Tired of Being Tired?

Powerful Multivitamin to Regain Energy and Vibrant Health

TERRY LEMEROND
JACOB TEITELBAUM, MD

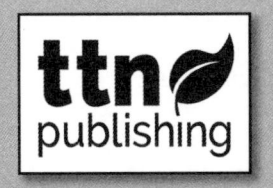

ttn publishing

Published by:
Terry Talks Nutrition Publishing
GREEN BAY, WI

The purpose of this book is to educate. It is not intended to serve as a replacement for professional medical advice. Any use of the information in this book is at the reader's discretion. This book is sold with the understanding that neither the publisher nor the authors have any liability or responsibility for any injury caused or alleged to be caused directly or indirectly by the information contained in this book. While every effort has been made to ensure accuracy, the book's contents should not be construed as medical advice. To obtain medical advice on your individual health needs, please consult a qualified healthcare practitioner.

Copyright © 2024 TTN Publishing, LLC, Green Bay, WI

All rights reserved. Except as permitted under the United States Copyright Act of 1976, no part of this publication in any format, electronic or physical, may be reproduced or distributed in any form or by any means, or stored in a database or retrieval system without the prior written permission of the publisher.

Library of Congress Cataloging-in-Publication Data is on file with the Library of Congress.

ISBN: 978-1-952507-64-9

Editor: Kathleen Barnes • kathleenbarnes.com
Cover: Jill Cashin
Interior: Gary A. Rosenberg • www.thebookcouple.com

Printed in the United States of America

10 9 8 7 6 5 4 3 2 1

Contents

Part 1: The Problem

1. You Need a Multivitamin. *Why?* 3
2. What's Wrong with Food? 13
3. Ridiculous(ly Low) Dietary Allowances (RDAs) 19

Part 2: What Do You Really Need?

4. Antioxidants: Even Humans Rust without These 25
5. The Critical Importance of B Vitamins 33
6. Vitamins D and K for Bone, Immune
   and Heart Health 41
7. Minerals 45
8. Amino Acids and More 59

Part 3: The Solution

9. What Proof Do We Have? 75
10. The Right Stuff 79

References 87
Index 91
About the Authors 97

PART 1

THE PROBLEM

CHAPTER 1

You Need a Multivitamin. *Why?*

We'll start this off unequivocally: If you're not taking a multivitamin every day—yes, every single day—you should be. Your life depends on it.

We hear the arguments against supplementation all the time.

Why should we take multivitamins? Our ancestors survived for millennia without them, right?

That's an excellent question and a valid one.

Our ancestors ate a whole food natural diet. There were no Cheetos or Cinnabons or Cokes. There were no pesticides or herbicides or newfangled factory farming techniques. Their food came quite literally hand to mouth. They harvested mushrooms and tubers in the woods, they hunted game and caught fish. For the most part, they ate what they harvested on the same day.

Our North American ancestors never ever ate pineapples transported by ship and truck from halfway around the world. They never ever ate baguettes from France or sugar-laden Mars bars from China. Their meat came from wild animals that never saw the inside of a pen or treatment with growth hormones to make them grow bigger and more profitable to factory farmers.

Our ancestors got their vitamins and minerals from wild harvesting and later from crops grown on soils that contained a wealth of nutrients and from wild animals.

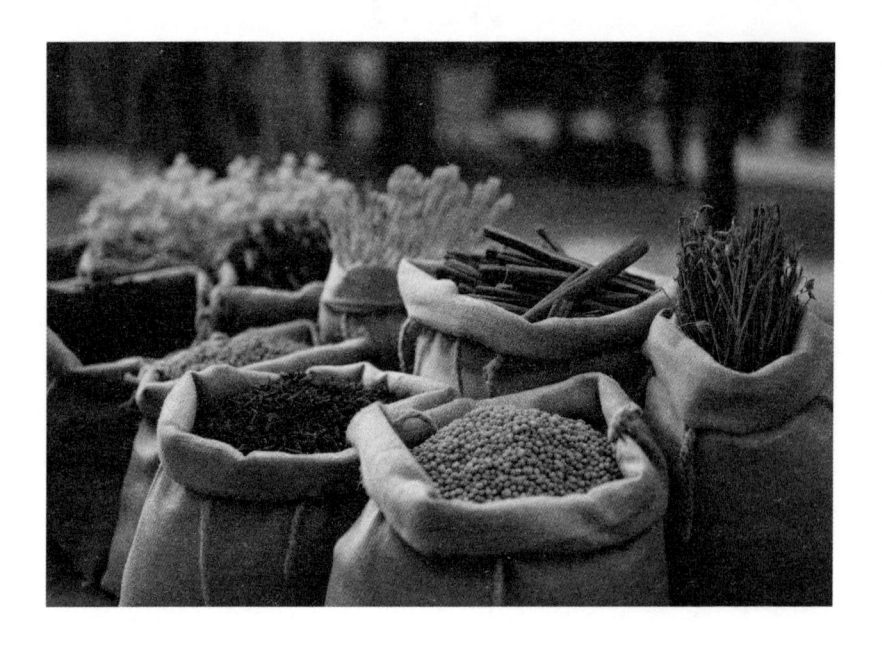

True, those same ancestors lived relatively short lives (about 33 years) compared to today's average North American lifespan of about 73 years. But that was then and now is now. Many prehistoric humans died in their first year of life. Ancient women frequently died in childbirth and accidents and wars surely took their toll and shortened their lives.

In today's world, we get an extra 40 years more than our ancestors on average, thanks at least in part to modern medicine that has given us antibiotics to ward off all types of infections, the ability to monitor pregnancy and childbirth in far safer ways, trauma medicine to handle accidents, modern plumbing instead of chamber pots and a vast array of medicines to ward off the diseases of aging.

Today, most of us zip back and forth from high-stress jobs, plop down in front of the TV at night with a bag of potato chips and a Coke, and celebrate on weekends with fat-laden meals and alcoholic beverages.

You can see where we're going here. In today's world of ultra-processed "food," we are fatter than ever and more malnourished than at any time in history. We need essential vitamins and minerals every day in order to build the strong, healthy bodies our modern world has denied us.

Nutritionally starved

Nutrient deficient soil produces nutrient deficient crops. Our food (produce and meat) comes mostly from factory farms where the soil has been depleted of vital nutrients, meaning we and animals raised on this land can no longer get those vital nutrients from food as we did from food produced in nutrient-rich soil.

Nutritional components of fruits, vegetables and grains grown in our North American soil have drastically decreased in the last 80 years. Intense mismanaged farming has decreased overall soil nutrients by 42 percent, phosphorus by 27 percent, and sulfur by 33 percent since 1950.

In a 2004 study, 43 garden crops were analyzed to compare nutritional content in 1950 versus 1999, using USDA data. Some nutrients were unchanged, but calcium, phosphorus, iron, riboflavin and vitamin C were all much lower in 1999 compared to 1950, ranging from a 6 percent to 38 percent drop.

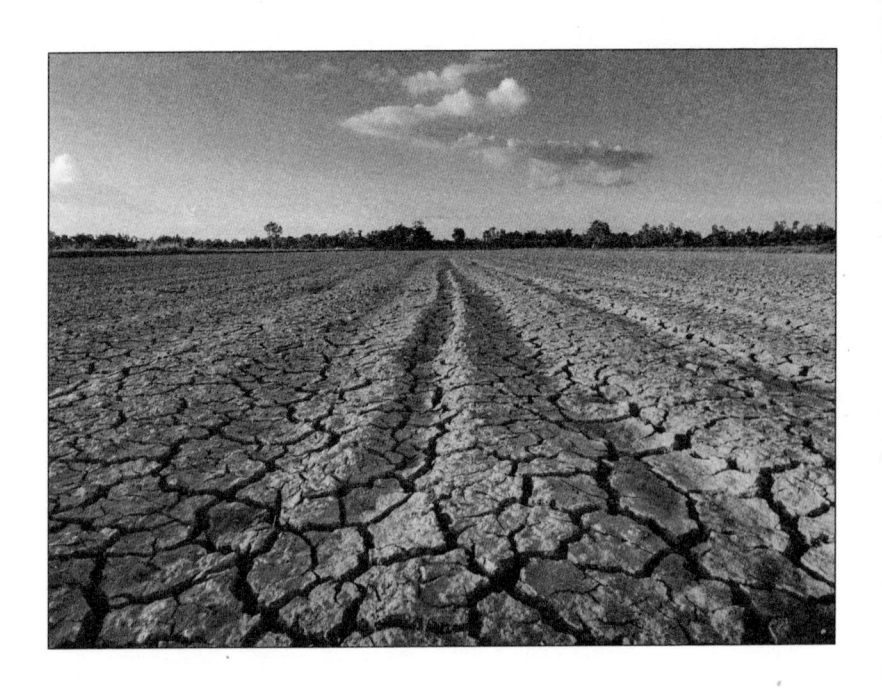

Additionally, pesticides and herbicides are broadly used to produce higher crop yields. These dangerous chemicals leave behind an array of toxic residues that cause endocrine disruption and cancer as well as contaminating the entire food chain.

So now we have these nutrient-depleted fruits, vegetables, grains and meats transported to the Big Food industry, which processes the heck out of them, robbing them of even more nutrients to the point where that unnaturally orange Cheeto you were just about to pop into your mouth has virtually no nutritional value. Zero. Plus, it has added chemicals including preservatives, additives and artificial colors that your body cannot use. Yuck!

The average American's diet today includes over 140 pounds of added sugar per year—18 percent of the average daily caloric intake with absolutely no nutritional value.

The added sugar alone makes the average American diet a disaster. Sugar also suppresses the immune system and stimulates yeast overgrowth in the intestines. Add in highly processed white flour and rice and we've reduced our vitamin and mineral intake by 35 percent. Now add to this the nutrients that are lost in the canning of vegetables and fruits, which can cause vitamin losses of up to 80 percent, and in the processing of other foods and the 42% lost to soil depletion, and the numbers make it clear: We're in the hole nutritionally. We're in trouble.

This, in our opinion, is the underlying cause of the obesity epidemic we are seeing in America and around the industrialized world. We are quite literally starving, and our nutrient-deprived brains are desperately seeking "food," turning to nutritionally void Skittles, Big Macs, Pepsis, anything we can grab to squelch our bodies' urgent demands for nutrition. The result: We gain weight, our bodies are starved, and we get sicker and sicker.

Tongue in cheek: Well, that's OK because we have pharmaceuticals to fight cancer and other diseases caused by toxic exposures. But we digress...

The Stress Monster

Now let's add in the stress monster. Yes, the stress of the modern-day world is a monster. All of us feel it, probably on a daily basis.

You slept through your alarm and had to rush to get kids' lunches and get them off to school, perhaps silently berating your spouse for not helping more, discovering your work deadline has been shortened without co-workers consulting with you, finding your car battery dead when you leave work, making you late to pick up your daughter from soccer practice, necessitating a trip to Mickey D's to pick up dinner, kids jittery and unwilling to go to bed after their huge dose of sugar and processed foods and finally, your turn to sleep, only you find yourself lying awake re-hashing the stressors of the day.

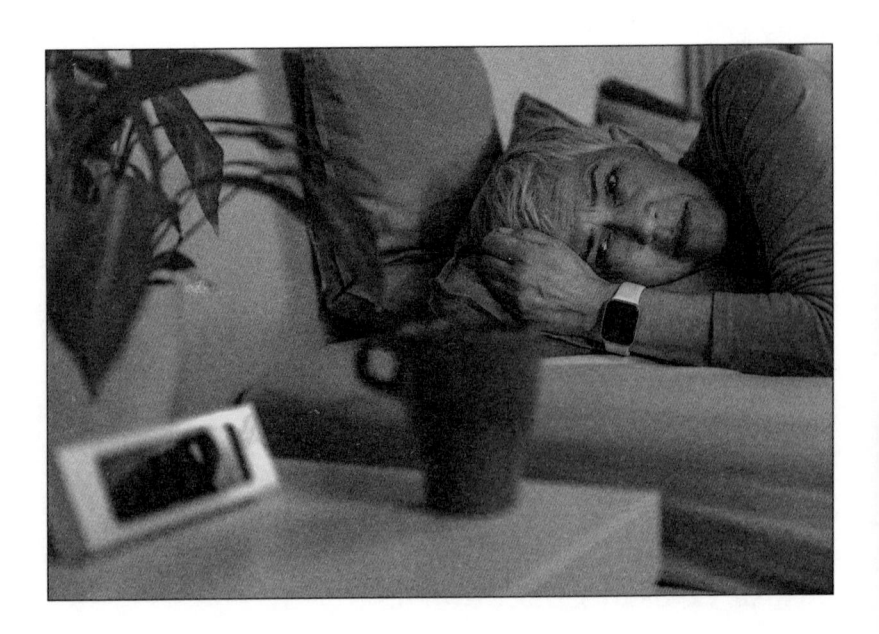

This has happened to every one of us.

Most of us don't address stress adequately or maybe we just learn to live with it. That's life, after all.

But stress takes its toll in many disease-causing ways. Australian researchers found that unrelieved emotional stress reduces levels of essential nutrients including magnesium, zinc, calcium, iron and niacin.

It's simple. We all need a powerhouse of vitamins and minerals to survive and thrive. If you've read this far, we're pretty sure you agree with us.

Let's take a few paragraphs to introduce ourselves and our personal journeys that give us the credentials to guide you to the multivitamin that will take care of almost all of your nutritional needs.

From Dr. Teitelbaum:

During medical school, a bout of post-viral chronic fatigue syndrome forced me to drop out. I was too sick to work, and I had been paying my own way. I found myself homeless and sleeping in parks.

I was crushed, convinced that everything I had worked for in my life was over. But the Universe had other plans for me. It was as if a cosmic "Holistic Homeless Medical School" sign magically appeared on my park bench.

At the time, I didn't even know there was such a thing as holistic healing. But naturopaths, herbalists, nutritionists and countless other holistic health practitioners wandered by my park bench. They taught me the bits and pieces of what I needed to learn to recover, return to medical school and get my honors in medicine.

I am very much a science geek and would often spend my nights going through the journal stacks in the medical library. I would find countless studies showing that natural remedies helped.

Surprised, I asked my medical school professors about them. But surprise, surprise! Most refused to look at the studies, saying that "it must all be pseudoscience," and that they had "never seen any studies showing natural remedies helped."

But a few of the skeptical professors and later my skeptical medical colleagues said, "That must be nonsense!" But some actually did look at the studies just to prove I was wrong. These doctors would usually come back several days later asking what other studies I had. They would often then go on to become holistic physicians.

I found my niche!

From Terry Lemerond:

When I was growing up, I was fortunate (or unfortunate) to have access to many things that weren't good for me. Junk food, candy and soft drinks became the major staples of my diet. As a young man of 20, I weighed over 200 pounds. At a height of 5'6", I was nearly as wide around as I was tall. I also had very severe hypoglycemia which resulted in a lot of mental, emotional and behavioral problems due to the constant mood swings caused by my erratically plummeting blood sugar levels.

I realized my life was in trouble and decided to join the Marine Corps to try to get myself on track. That's when I met Captain Ed Vito. This amazing man took me under his wing and helped me learn the value of good health and proper nutrition. With his guidance, I became healthier and happier. My mood swings disappeared, and I felt better about life than I ever had before. When I returned to Green Bay after my stint in the Marines, people didn't recognize the man I had become.

I was extremely excited about what healthy food, good nutrition, and vitamins could do and quickly started learning everything I could on the subjects. I got a job at the only health food store in town, worked every chance I got and eventually became owner of the business. Through years of study and experience, a dream grew in my heart: to create a company that would develop and sell state-of-the-art nutritional and botanical products. I went on to start Enzymatic Therapy, a company I ran for 20 years and eventually sold, and I am currently founder and president of EuroPharma, where I introduced the Terry Naturally and EuroMedica line of products to help people improve their health, and Terry Naturally Animal Health to improve the health of pets. I feel incredibly blessed to be able to inspire and help others live a life of vibrant health and happiness. I've also shared what I've learned with the public through my website, radio show, blog and more at Terry Talks Nutrition (https://terrytalksnutrition.com/).

In Conclusion...

The Standard American Diet (SAD) has left Americans nutritionally starved. High-quality multivitamins are the answers. In this book, we'll guide you to the right choices in the confusing world of nutritional supplements.

CHAPTER 2

What's Wrong with Food?

What's wrong with food? Absolutely nothing!

Food is the stuff of life. As much as the nutritional value of our food supply has diminished in recent decades, for the reasons we reviewed in Chapter 1, food must still *always* be our Number 1 source of nutrition.

We're sorry if you thought you could subsist on the Big Mac diet and pop a couple of capsules to make up for any nutritional shortfalls. Nice try!

No. Just no.

Even the perfect multivitamin should be considered an insurance policy, not a substitute for a healthy eating plan.

SAD, so sad

In general, the Standard American Diet (SAD) is a disaster. It's astronomically high in empty calories, sugar, refined grains (white flour), saturated fat, red meat and salt. In addition, the convenience foods we pick up in the grocery store or at our local fast-food joints (and even restaurants) contain a slew of chemicals and added sugar and salt (sodium).

It's fair to say that our busy modern lifestyle makes it easy for us to rely on easy and quick foods. These are precisely the foods that are destroying our health. Lacking in vitamins, minerals and fiber, this eating pattern sets us up for chronic diseases based on inflammation, oxidation and toxic exposure. More about that in a few pages, but let's start now with the concept that we are a nation of overweight people who are literally starving for the nutrition our bodies crave.

Here are some sobering numbers:

* We're getting heavier and heavier. According to the Centers for Disease Control and Prevention (CDC), an astonishing 74% of American adults are overweight. Compare that to a 44.8% prevalence of overweight in 1960.

* In the 1960s, roughly 13% of American adults were considered obese. Today, just 60 years later, that figure has more than *tripled* to 43%!

* Severe obesity (called morbid obesity) has increased by *tenfold* in the same time period with 10% of American adults weighing 100 pounds or more above their ideal body weight.

* Add in children and the obesity statistics become truly frightening, affecting 15% of children under the age of 18 today, triple the 5% rate in the 1960s.

* And it's getting worse: 22% of children over 12 are considered obese today.

The whys

So, here's the obvious question: Why are these numbers escalating at such an alarming rate?

Here's a simple answer: We are starving. Our bodies are craving the nutrients we so desperately need. Our brains keep sending out signals that say, "Eat! Eat! I'm starving." (It's actually a hormone called leptin that sends out these signals, but that's probably more than you want to know right now.)

Yes, indeed, we are starving. We need vitamin B12, the B complex energy vitamins, iron, zinc and a host of other vitamins and minerals that our SAD denies us. We need fiber, found in whole grains, vegetables and fruits, not pizza, hotdogs, sodas and fries.

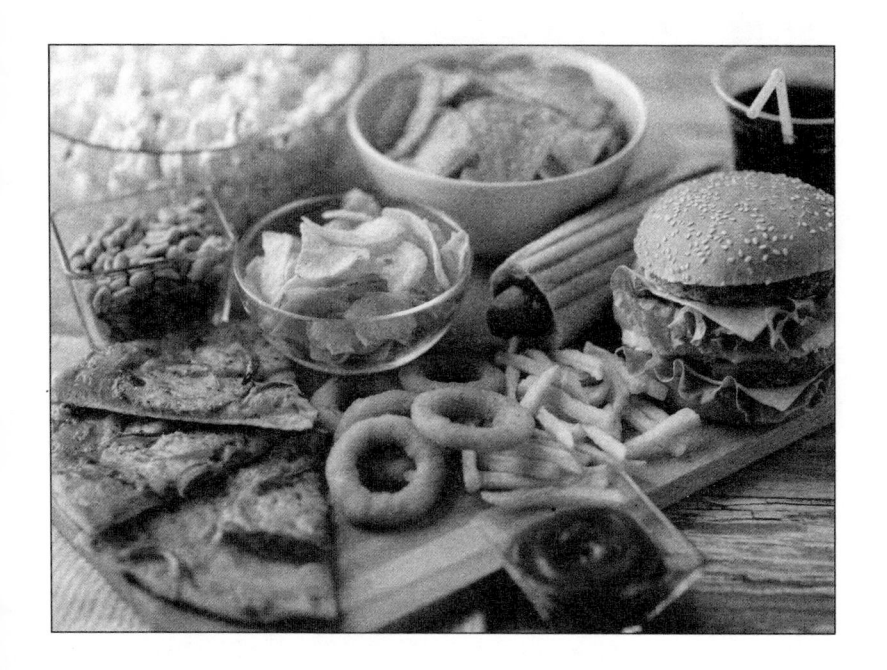

The wherefores

Clearly not all of us are overweight. However, unless you are super vigilant about your food intake, you've probably slid into the SAD nightmare, no matter whether you are overweight or not. Have you even noticed that when you indulge in a fast-food meal, you crave more? Or how terrible it tastes if you haven't given in to those cravings for a few weeks? Yes, these things are addictive, probably quite intentionally.

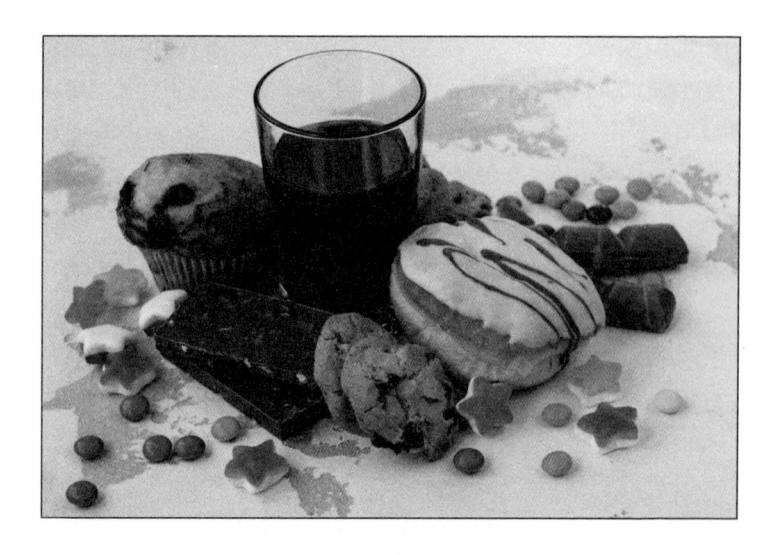

Yes, the main players in fast food hell—MSG, refined flour, high fructose corn syrup and gluten—actually "hijack" your brain and tell your pancreas to release more insulin, making you feel hungrier, according to Harvard nutritionists.

All of this adds up to an epidemic of heart disease, type 2 diabetes, cancer, dementia and more. It's not pretty.

What's Wrong with Food?

Our nutrient deficit

Remember the good old days when the US Department of Agriculture recommended five servings of fruits and vegetables a day? Now they say we need at least nine servings. That's a pretty strong indicator of our nutritional shortfalls in itself. Sadly, only about 10% of us even get five a day, according to the American Heart Association. Wow. That's pretty mind boggling!

BTW, French fries don't count.

Yet numerous studies show us that an intake of five to nine servings of fruits and vegetables daily is the strongest contributor to longevity.

Add all of this into the nutrient loss in our soils and resulting lower nutritional value in our produce we outlined in Chapter 1, and you'll see how difficult it has become to get every single nutrient you need even with a stellar diet rich in fruits, vegetables, healthy fats and proteins.

We won't say it is impossible to get every nutrient from food in order to remain healthy for a lifetime, but it's certainly extremely difficult.

Here's where your multivitamin comes in.

We can't emphasize strongly enough that your focus should be on food as your primary source of nutrients, but a multivitamin will fill in the gaps where nutritional shortfalls are inevitable, since it will supply optimal levels of key nutrients, beyond what the SAD can do.

Stay with us. There are answers.

SMOOTHIE RECIPE

Want to guarantee your 9-A-Day? Here's a simple way—if you have a decent blender.

Blend up the following for 2–3 minutes to ensure a smooth texture:

- 1 cup spinach or kale
- ½ cup carrots
- ½ bell pepper
- ¼ cup celery
- 1 small orange
- A handful of other fruit, including berries, cherries, pineapple, etc. (Frozen is OK and makes the drink cold.)
- Enough water for a drinkable liquid. Ice cubes are fine, too.

Feel free to add your multivitamin powder to this nutritional powerhouse.

Organic produce is preferable as much as possible.

Feel free to get creative!

Think about this: This super smoothie gives you seven servings of fruits and veggies. If you add a salad at lunchtime and a veggie or even two at dinner, you've surpassed the 9-A-Day mark and supercharged your nutrient intake.

CHAPTER 3

Ridiculous(ly Low) Dietary Allowances (RDAs)

The government, in its great wisdom, has decided that its Recommended Dietary Allowances (RDAs) are the levels of intake of essential nutrients that are judged by the Food and Nutrition Board to be adequate to meet the known nutrient needs of practically all healthy persons.

In simple terms, this means that the government is delineating a bare minimum intake of vitamins and minerals to prevent serious disease in "practically all healthy persons."

Did you notice what we call "weasel words?" Maybe it's just governmentspeak, but there is no such thing as "practically all healthy persons."

We are all different. In scientific terms, this is called "bioindividuality." There is no one else on Earth who has the identical genetics, health conditions and toxic environmental exposures, not even if you are an identical twin. That means your nutritional needs can't be put into a simple box.

Those Recommended Dietary Allowances or what

Dr. Teitelbaum calls "Ridiculous(ly low) Dietary Allowances" are based on what is needed to prevent diseases of deficiency, like beriberi (thiamine deficiency), rickets (vitamin D deficiency) and scurvy (vitamin C deficiency), not on what is OPTIMAL.

We prefer the best.

In addition, higher levels of most nutrients are often needed to compensate for poor absorption of nutrients due to several causes including everyday stress, illness, even taking PPI (protein pump inhibitor) acid blockers.

Let's take a look at vitamin C. Virtually all scientists agree that vitamin C is essential to human health. So, what does the RDA say about our needs? The RDA says that adult men need 90 mg a day and women need 75 mg a day.

That's just enough vitamin C to prevent scurvy, characterized by rotting teeth and gums, anemia, bone and joint pain and depression. That is not the most desirable intake by any stretch of the imagination.

If you eat an orange every single day (who does?), you'll be getting about 70 mg of vitamin C. That's not enough, even by the RDA levels. Please keep in mind that we're also talking about diminished nutrients in our food supply due to soil depletion that we talked about in Chapter 2, and our apparent growing national aversion to fresh whole food.

Of course, vitamin C is just one essential nutrient. A great multivitamin should include at least 13 key vitamins, 9 minerals and 5 amino acids.

What do we really need? After nearly a century (that's right) of research on human nutrient needs between the two of us, we should aim for 250 mg of vitamin C a day. That's more than three times the amount the government says women need and 278% more than the RDA for men. That would be 3.5 oranges. Or a supplement.

We've just used vitamin C as an example here, but it's important for you to know that (it's worth repeating) we all need at least 13 key vitamins, 9 minerals and 5 amino acids every day. The RDA for virtually every single one falls far short of optimal.

What vitamins and minerals do you need? In short, by definition, all of them are essential and can't be made effectively by our bodies.

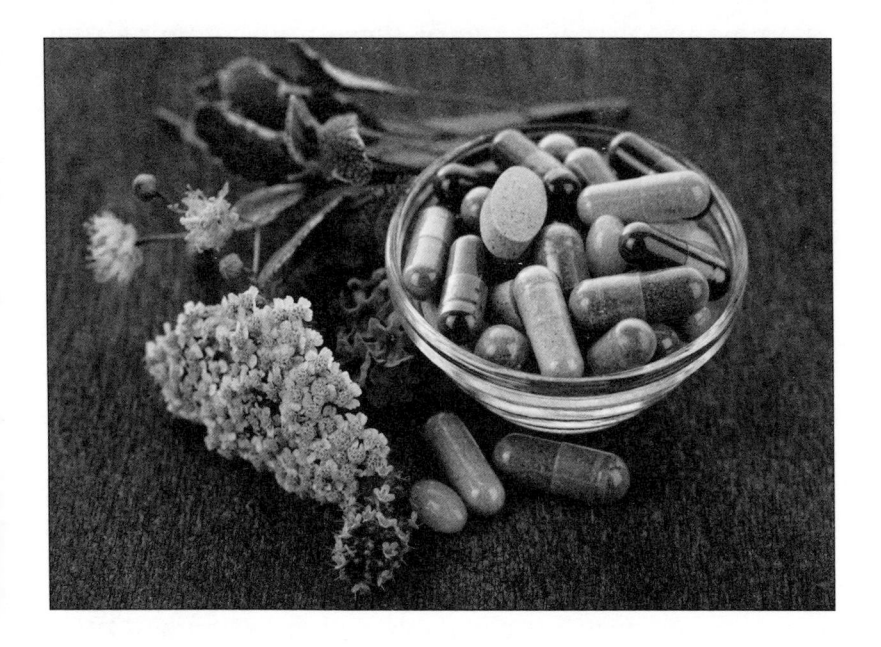

Each nutrient is critical to health, and it is helpful to understand the roles they play. In the coming chapters, you'll find a "Nutrition Primer" that reviews the key nutrients you should be getting from your diet, and the optimal amounts. Looking at this research, it will be very clear that the government's RDAs are not ideal for many nutrients.

Don't panic though! We will also show you how to get all of these easily without being part of the "Handful Club" where you take handfuls of supplements all day!

Here's a little mind-bending argument against popping dozens of pills: Frequently they are not absorbed as they pass through your digestive tract. The port-a-potty cleanout folks can attest to this. I'll leave the rest to your imagination, but let it suffice to say that there is ample proof that many of these multivitamins pass through the human digestive tract almost completely undissolved.

It'll be a relief for you to hear that all of the key micronutrients you should get from your diet can be obtained in one simple nutritional drink daily. Except for iron, which is toxic if you are not deficient; calcium, which blocks thyroid hormone absorption and which most people do not need (contrary to sales hype); digestive enzymes and omega fatty acids (fats and water don't mix); you can get all you need from one simple drink.

Best of all, the right powdered multivitamin added to plain water, or even mixed into your favorite smoothie, can give you all the key vitamins, minerals and amino acids you need easily, affordably and digestibly at OPTIMAL levels!

PART 2

WHAT DO YOU REALLY NEED?

Ready to learn what is best? For each nutrient we give a range. For example:

MAGNESIUM

Recommended daily dosage: 100–200 mg

The higher number is what would be in one daily scoop of a high-quality multivitamin powder. But if cost or a sensitive stomach are issues, you can take half a scoop a day (the lower number) and still get amazing nutritional support for each nutrient!

CHAPTER 4

Antioxidants: Even Humans Rust without These

We've all heard of vitamins, and probably most of our readers know something about individual vitamins. But have you heard of antioxidants?

Anti = against, oxidants = oxygen? Against oxygen? Isn't that counterintuitive? Don't we need oxygen to live?

Yes, of course, we need oxygen to breathe, but oxygen in the wrong place, especially within our cells, creates toxic little troublemakers called free radical oxygen species (ROS). These unstable atoms are often caused by exposure to environmental toxins like air pollutants, cigarette smoke, ozone and industrial chemicals, damaging our cells, causing disease and accelerating aging.

Yes, the immune system can vacuum up free radicals and neutralize them up to a point, but our modern world continuously assaults our immune systems, so sometimes they break down.

Additionally, we need to adapt to an environment where new infections are coming to the surface. This back-and-forth between humans and microorganisms has been going on throughout history, with both sides developing new weapons and defenses.

Our immune system is dependent on key antioxidant nutrients, such as zinc and vitamin A, to function.

In addition to being critical for energy production, antioxidants are also essential for maintaining health and youth. In fact, doctors who specialize in "anti-aging medicine" use antioxidants (as well as bioidentical hormones) as key tools. Why? Oxidation is the same thing that happens when something rusts. Antioxidants help keep our body young.

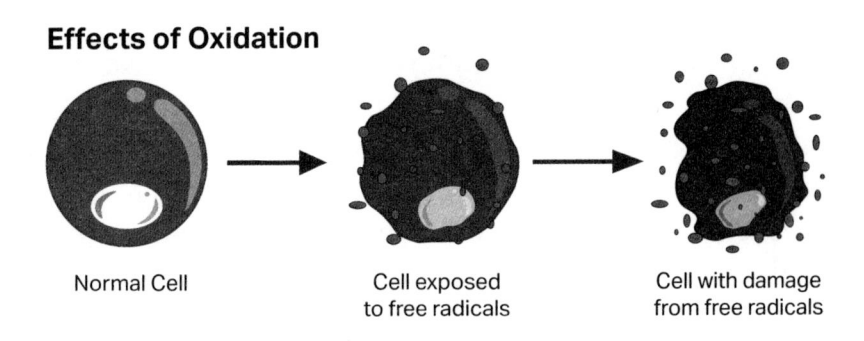

Effects of Oxidation

Normal Cell → Cell exposed to free radicals → Cell with damage from free radicals

Antioxidants Made by Our Bodies

Supplemental antioxidant nutrients from plants and other sources are extremely popular, and for good reason. But we feel that the first emphasis should be placed on the two antioxidants that our bodies produce on their own:

Glutathione. This is the most critical antioxidant, serving countless functions. Deficiency is very common, especially in people chronically using acetaminophen (Tylenol). It plays key roles in:

* Detoxification
* Protecting the body from disease causing inflammation
* Regulating cell division and protection from cancer
* Improving insulin sensitivity
* Guarding against fatty liver and other liver disease
* Helping improve health conditions including Parkinson's disease, ulcerative colitis and eye diseases.

Super oxide dismutase (SOD). Deficiency of this is rare if people are getting zinc and a little bit of copper. Unfortunately, inflammatory and infectious conditions that are so common today can cause massive zinc losses, setting us up to be the victims of our own inflammatory processes.

Plenty of zinc and a little copper can help your body make abundant amounts of your own SOD and give you protection against:

* cancer
* inflammatory diseases
* cystic fibrosis
* artery blockages
* premature aging
* rheumatoid arthritis
* neurodegenerative diseases
* diabetes

How do we optimize production of glutathione and SOD for daily health? It can be done easily by starting with N-Acetyl Cysteine, other key antioxidants and some essential vitamins.

NAC (N-ACETYL CYSTEINE)

Recommended daily dosage: 125–250 mg

NAC is critical for making glutathione and for keeping vitamins C and E in their active forms. Although taking most forms of glutathione by mouth has no effect on blood levels (it simply gets oxidized and digested), taking NAC and glycine, the key amino acid "building blocks" of glutathione (plus vitamin C), can markedly increase glutathione levels. Food sources include eggs, meat, fish, dairy products and seeds.

For most people's day-to-day needs, having NAC in their multivitamin powder is the way to go.

NAC has other benefits as well, perhaps because it helps raise glutathione.

In one study, taking high dose NAC improved the time to muscle fatigue by 30% while preventing a drop in glutathione and can even help to protect the heart muscle during a heart attack.

NAC at much higher doses (600–3,000 mg/day) even significantly decreased symptoms of OCD (obsessive compulsive disorder) and other psychological disorders.

NAC also helps your body get rid of toxins, while protecting cells and keeping your body young.

Benefits of Other Nutritional Antioxidants

Antioxidants protect your body in many other ways as well. One clinical study found that men taking low-dose antioxidants were 1/3 less likely to have died of any cause by the end of the study. As just a few of many other examples, antioxidants such as vitamin C can decrease the hearing and vision loss that accompanies aging. Antioxidants also protect against stomach cancer, help in the treatment of liver disease, are associated with a decreased risk of hip fractures, and may protect against strokes.

VITAMIN C

Recommended daily dosage: 125–250 mg.

Scurvy, a nasty disease caused by vitamin C deficiency, is starting to make a comeback in the US. A study from the University of Arizona and published in the *American Journal of Public Health,* found that men and women aged 25 to 44 often fail to take in adequate amounts of vitamin C and are at high risk of getting scurvy.

Because the disease is seldom considered by 21st century healthcare practitioners, people presenting with scurvy symptoms such as fatigue, bleeding gums, or swollen extremities are often misdiagnosed and medicated for other disorders.

Vitamin C is already well known as a critical nutrient for proper immune, adrenal and antioxidant function, so we won't spend much time on it.

As extra encouragement, did you know that low vitamin C in the bloodstream correlates with increased body fat and waist measurements? Nutrition researchers from Arizona State University report that the amount of vitamin C in the bloodstream directly improves fat oxidation—the body's ability to use fat as a fuel source—during both exercise and at rest.

Vitamin C has been shown to prevent osteoporosis and may protect against developing angina (chest pain that may indicate heart stress) or strokes.

Vitamin C does make you less likely to catch a cold. In one study, people taking 500 mg of vitamin C a day had 18% fewer colds than those in the 50 mg/day group.

Vitamin C also helps improve sperm count and sperm motility and can be helpful in treating infertility.

VITAMIN E

Recommended daily dosage: 37–75 IU of mixed tocopherols

This critical antioxidant serves many functions, but more is not always better. Many nutrients (such as beta carotene) are part of a larger "family," so taking very high doses of only one type can suppress the others and become problematic.

To make this easier to understand, think of a category called "silverware." If you ordered a thousand knives and put them in your silverware drawer, you suddenly would not be able to find the forks and spoons. Scientists call this a "relative deficiency."

This is the case with vitamin E, which has many family members, called tocopherols. Research suggests that taking over 100 units of vitamin E a day can be problematic, increasing the risk of cancer and other problems.

This is because most supplements use only one member of the vitamin E family—alpha-tocopherol.

Taking only one out of a large family of vitamin Es can make people deficient in all the other forms. Because of this, we recommend taking 75 units a day as the ideal level in multivitamins. Better yet? The best multivitamin would use a blend of many different types of vitamin E, known as mixed tocopherols.

Although more of vitamin E is not better, deficiency is a significant problem. For example, research suggests that 91% of 2- to 5-year-olds are vitamin E deficient. Taking vitamin E (200 units twice a day—but only use a mixed tocopherol at these high doses) can also significantly reduce the severity and duration of menstrual period pain. Vitamin E in optimal doses (75 units a day) may also be cancer protective. For example, high blood levels of vitamin E cut the risk of prostate cancer by about 50 percent, and another study showed that vitamin E caused prostate cancer cells to "self-destruct."

Adequate vitamin E may also decrease the risk of breast cancer.

Given the above, one could argue that you'd need to be demented not to get adequate antioxidant support. It's not surprising that in a study on 1,033 people aged 65 years and older, low plasma levels of vitamin E were found to be associated with a more than doubled risk of becoming demented and of suffering from cognitive impairment!

Food sources of vitamin E include wheat germ, sunflower and safflower oil, almonds, peanuts and green leafy vegetables.

VITAMIN A

Recommended daily dosage:
750–1,500 mcg vitamin A as retinol

Vitamin A, an antioxidant found in abundance in green leafy vegetables, carrots, dairy products and fish, is critical for immunity and zinc function. But be careful to get the right type and not to get too much. High dosages can cause birth defects and osteoporosis.

Beta carotene, a form of vitamin A, is the main type used in most supplements because it is cheap. Unfortunately, at higher levels, some studies suggest beta carotene may cause cancer.

Retinol is the safer and much more effective form of vitamin A, when recommended doses are used.

For example, a large study looking at over 500,000 million "person years" showed that higher levels of dietary vitamin A intake were associated with a 17–32% lower risk of dying of any cause compared to those who did not get sufficient amounts of A.

Specifically, optimized retinol intake was associated with lower overall mortality, including death from stroke, heart and respiratory diseases.

Other benefits of vitamin A? They are too numerous to go into in detail, but younger skin, less acne and a healthy immune system are just a few.

CHAPTER 5

The Critical Importance of B Vitamins

B vitamins convert the food you eat into energy as well as a host of other critical functions. These include being essential for nerve, brain and immune function and much more. The government's RDAs (Ridiculous Dietary Allowances) are exceptionally low.

Food sources of these essential nutrients include nuts, legumes (dried beans and peas), whole grains, meat, fish, dairy products and some vitamin B12 fortified cereals.

VITAMIN B1 (THIAMINE)

Recommended daily dosage: (25–50 mg)

You need vitamin B1 for proper brain function, making it especially important in those with "brain fog." It is also critical for heart function. Thiamine deficiency is a major contributor to congestive heart failure (CHF).

This easy treatment is often ignored, despite the fact that 33 percent of CHF patients are low in thiamine. Thiamine is also helpful in treating dementia, anxiety, neuropathy, fatigue, alcoholism, confusion, depression, pain, memory loss and balance issues.

Professor Michael Gold also found that people with Alzheimer's disease also have lower serum thiamine levels than those with other types of dementia.

In a double-blind study by Dr. David Benton, an expert on thiamine, supplementation with vitamin B1 improved mood, possibly by increasing synthesis of acetylcholine, a brain chemical associated with memory. Learning disorders as well as behavioral problems in young children (sometimes to the point of hospitalization) can improve with high dose thiamine treatment. Thiamine intake may also decrease risk of sudden infant death syndrome (SIDS).

VITAMIN B2 (RIBOFLAVIN)

Recommended daily dosage: 75 mg

This B vitamin is especially critical for energy production. In higher doses (75–400 mg/day) it has been repeatedly shown to decrease migraine frequency by 67% after 6 to 12 weeks. Vitamin B2 even helps decrease the risk of postpartum depression.

Although Dr. Teitelbaum often starts people with migraines at a much higher dose, 75 mg a day as part of a daily multivitamin is sufficient for maintaining the benefits of this important B vitamin.

VITAMIN B3 (NIACIN)

Recommended daily dosage: 25–50 mg

Niacin is critical for energy production and may also prevent Alzheimer's disease.

A five-year study of more than 3,700 people showed that those who took more niacin had a lower risk of both Alzheimer's disease and age-related mental decline. The group getting a median 14 mg of niacin daily from diet (found in peanuts, avocados, brown rice, tuna and more) and supplements were at highest risk (current RDA for niacin is 16 mg per day for men and 14 mg per day for women).

While some benefits were noted with a lower amount of 17 mg per day, a daily niacin intake of 45 mg offered the most protection from Alzheimer's disease and other causes of cognitive decline.

But more is not better. Too high of an intake may lead to damage to blood vessels, and very high levels—over 1,000 mg daily—can increase diabetes and liver inflammation risk. We recommend the mixed niacin and niacinamide form, as higher doses of regular niacin can cause flushing (temporary, harmless reddening of the skin).

VITAMIN B5 (PANTOTHENIC ACID)

Recommended daily dosage: 50–100 mg

The B5 family is important in over 70 different functions in the body, including:

* Proper adrenal function—suspect adrenal fatigue if you get irritable when hungry ("hangry")
* Carbohydrate metabolism
* Metabolism of proteins
* Making healthy new blood cells

* Making acetylcholine, the brain chemical critical for memory
* Detoxification
* Protecting against vascular disease

VITAMIN B6 (PYRIDOXINE)

Recommended daily dosage: 12.5–25 mg

Vitamin B6 serves many critical functions, including enhancing immune function and possibly decreasing the risk of heart disease and colon cancer. Deficiency can lead to cognitive impairment, irritability, depression, nerve pain, finger swelling and carpal tunnel syndrome.

Doses over 45 mg a day can worsen nerve pain (neuropathy), but this can be avoided by using the pyridoxal-5-phosphate (P-5-P) form of vitamin B6. This form also bypasses blocks in metabolism that may be resistant to regular forms of vitamin B6.

VITAMIN B7 (BIOTIN)

Recommended daily dosage: 100–200 mcg

Biotin is important for healthy hair, skin and nails.

VITAMIN B9 (FOLATE)

Recommended daily dosage: 170–340 mcg of activated 5-MTHF folate

Folate is critical for energy and red blood cell production, brain health and immune function. But in many illnesses, the body loses the ability to use regular folate.

To the rescue? A super preactivated form of 5-Methyltetrahydrofolate (5-MTHF) can turn your energy back on!

This can sometimes cause detoxification, a good sign of healing. If you're feeling uncomfortable when detoxifying, it is okay to lower the dose of whatever you are using to a comfortable level. Then slowly increase the dosage as your body gets back into balance and you feel more comfortable.

Folate protects against serious neural tube birth defects that develop in the earliest weeks of pregnancy. Doctors recommend that women who are pregnant or trying to get pregnant take a vitamin supplement that includes folate to prevent birth defects and other complications.

Interestingly, since food manufacturers began adding extra folate to flour in 1998 to prevent birth defects, we have seen that the rates of heart disease, stroke, blood pressure, colon cancer and osteoporosis have all fallen. Researchers are now advocating that the current fortification level, 140 micrograms of folate per 100 grams of grain, should be doubled.

Folate also helps:

* Increase bone strength
* Improve memory and prevent Alzheimer's disease
* Lower blood pressure and risk of stroke
* Decrease risk of ovarian cancer
* Ease depression

VITAMIN B12 (COBALAMIN)

Recommended daily dosage: 250–500 mcg of methylcobalamin

Vitamin B12 is a key nutrient that works in tandem with folic acid to strengthen bones, while decreasing the risk of stroke and breast cancer, especially in postmenopausal women.

Dr. Teitelbaum has found that treating patients with vitamin B12, even if their levels are technically normal, often results in marked energy and mental improvement. This is good, as Vitamin B12 is both very safe and cheap—even in high doses.

Absorption of B12 can be low due to many common situations, including:

1. Vegan diets. While these can be very healthy diets, B12 is more abundant in dairy products and meat.

2. Acid blocker medicines called PPIs (like omeprazole and other medications ending in "-prazole"). These medications are unnecessarily toxic, conservatively

contributing to over 30,000 US deaths a year, plus millions of cases of dementia and osteoporosis.

3. Low stomach acid, which is also a major cause of indigestion symptoms, especially in elderly people.
4. The diabetes medication metformin is an excellent medicine, but routinely causes B12 deficiency.

B VITAMINS AND THE "PERFECT STORM" FOR A HUMAN ENERGY CRISIS

Most Americans don't have the energy they would like, and research shows that 31% of adults have such severe fatigue that they consider it to be disabling. In fact, the American lifestyle is triggering "the perfect storm" for a human energy crisis of major proportions. Why?

* Approximately 50% of vitamins, minerals and other key nutrients (except the calories) are destroyed in food processing.
* The average night's sleep until 150 years ago, when light bulbs were invented, was nine hours a night. We are now down to 6¾ hours, a whopping 30% pay cut to our body.
* The speed and stress of human life is increasing.
* Hormonal problems triggered by stress.

CHAPTER 6

Vitamins D and K for Bone, Immune and Heart Health

VITAMIN D (CHOLECALCIFEROL)

Recommended daily dosage:
500–1,000 IU (12.5 -25 mcg) of vitamin D3

Vitamin D is arguably the most critical vitamin deficiency in the US. Our dropping levels cause an estimated 85,500 extra cancer deaths in the US each year. This shortfall is directly related to the deadly recommendation to avoid sun exposure.

The proper advice? Avoid sunburn, not sunshine!

A review in the *Mayo Clinic Proceedings* showed that 36% of healthy young adults and 57% of people in hospitals in the United States have inadequate levels of vitamin D. Vitamin D deficiency is especially common in people with chronic pain.

Sun exposure accounts for 90% of our vitamin D. What's not to love? It's free for everyone! It's also found in fatty fish and eggs.

Allow Dr. Teitelbaum to engage in a brief rant against a medical profession that mysteriously decided to warn against the dangers of sun exposure a few decades back, leading to the current widespread vitamin D deficiency.

> "This misguided advice, given to decrease the number of dangerous skin cancers called melanomas, is ludicrous. Why? Most melanomas are not in sun exposed areas (they are under our clothes). The skin cancers usually caused by sunshine (e.g. basal cell cancers) are usually quite benign. But many other deadly types of cancer increase in the face of vitamin D deficiency.
>
> For example, ideal amounts of vitamin D are important to minimize breast cancer risk.
>
> Ironically, the research has shown that avoiding sunshine (low Vitamin D) also makes melanomas *more* deadly!"

Dr. Edward Giovannucci, a Harvard University Professor of Medicine and Nutrition, suggests that adequate vitamin D intake might help prevent 30 deaths for each death caused by skin cancer.

"I would challenge anyone to find an area or nutrient or any factor that has such consistent anticancer benefits as vitamin D," Giovannucci told cancer scientists. "The data are really quite remarkable."

An intake of 2,000 units per day of vitamin D (through a mix of sunshine, food and supplements) could decrease both breast cancer and colon cancer by over 50%. In addition, higher vitamin D levels may slow the progression of breast cancer.

Vitamin D deficiency contributes to:

* Hip fractures and osteoporosis (weak bones)
* Multiple sclerosis
* Rheumatoid arthritis
* Diabetes
* Asthma
* Heart disease and hypertension
* Inflammatory bowel disease

Why do we have 500–1,000 IU (12.5–25 mcg) as the optimal level and not higher? For people with several health conditions, including chronic fatigue syndrome, fibromyalgia, long COVID and some autoimmune conditions, too much Vitamin D can convert to a form that is not picked up on blood testing, but blocks healthy immunity. So, in general, more may not be better. If needed, additional vitamin D can be dosed separately.

The dose above is what we consider the "sweet spot" for most people.

VITAMIN K2 (MENAQUINONE)

Recommended daily dosage: 50–100 mcg of MK7 menaquinone

Vitamin K, found in green leafy vegetables, broccoli, dairy products and fermented foods, has many important functions within the body. More are still being discovered.

Research has shown that vitamin K is an anticancer, bone strengthening and insulin-sensitizing molecule.

In a study of over 50,000 people, low dietary vitamin K intake was associated with a 14 to 21% higher risk of hospitalization with heart attack related conditions.

A unique form of vitamin K2, called menaquinone, has been shown to help to reverse arterial stiffness of vessels going to the heart and brain.

The evidence suggests it may also decrease the risk of dementia, Parkinson's disease and other neurological conditions, neuropathy, migraines, and ... well, you get the picture. This is an exploding area of vitamin benefits research!

Vitamin K at this dose does *not* counteract the blood thinning effect of the prescription drug Coumadin (warfarin). Research shows that these *low* doses of vitamin K make the use of Coumadin safer, especially in people with difficulty controlling bleeding. Of course, if you're on Coumadin, get your doctor's OK before adding any supplement.

In conclusion...

We've just given you the briefest summary of the importance of essential vitamins. The comprehensive details and scientific research could fill an old-style encyclopedia, but it should be more than enough to show the importance of getting the right nutrients every day, in optimal forms, without the hassle of gulping handfuls of pills.

CHAPTER 7

Minerals

Minerals are just as important as vitamins in your overall health picture. Some are antioxidants, some help deal with endocrine challenges (like type 2 diabetes and hypothyroidism) and others are essential to wound healing, brain function, cancer prevention and much more.

Here's a brief list of essential minerals:

- Boron
- Magnesium
- Molybdenum
- Copper
- Iodine
- Selenium
- Chromium
- Manganese
- Zinc

If you're paying close attention, you've probably noticed that three well-known minerals, calcium, potassium and sodium are not included in this list from which we'll concoct our perfect multivitamin.

WHAT WE DON'T NEED AND WHY

Although the Standard American Diet (SAD) loses about 50% of key minerals in food processing, there are two minerals that we get plenty of:

* **Sodium:** Salt, a/k/a sodium chloride, is the biggest source of sodium in the SAD. If you're breaking out of the box and creating your meals from fresh whole food, feel free to use your salt grinder to taste. Processed food contains excessive amounts of salt (and sugar) to cover up the taste of the garbage that comes out of the other end in food processing, so avoid processed foods as much as possible. Salt supplementation should take place at your table, not in some factory, preferably with sea salt. The problem with sea salt is that it is low in iodine, but a great multivitamin will have just the right amount of iodine and other key minerals.

* **Calcium:** We are not a calcium-deficient society, thanks to our addiction to cheese and other calcium-rich dairy products. In fact, even for osteoporosis (loss of bone density), calcium supplementation has minimal benefit. What does help increase bone density? Nutrients such as boron, magnesium, vitamin D and others, which your multivitamin should contain. Calcium is not heart healthy, and also blocks thyroid hormone absorption, so it's best to keep levels low in a multivitamin.

* **Potassium:** Unfortunately, there is one critical mineral that the government simply does not allow to be added to a multivitamin in meaningful amounts, so it cannot be included. This is potassium, which is important for preventing high blood pressure. Potassium can be easily obtained by drinking tomato and other vegetable juices or eating avocados or bananas.

MAGNESIUM

Recommended daily dosage: 100–200 mg

Magnesium is probably one of the best-known minerals and one that is especially essential for life. It is found in a wide variety of foods, but there are critical nutritional deficiencies in our modern diet.

Put simply, magnesium deficiency is common and is one of the most critical nutritional problems we face.

Magnesium is involved in over 600 different body functions, but many of us have low magnesium levels because minerals are lost in food processing. The average American diet supplies 245 milligrams of magnesium per day, while the average Asian diet supplies over 600 milligrams per day.

The best supplementation amount is 200 mg daily. That is lower than the Ridiculous(ly low) Daily Allowance (RDA). Here's why:

Higher levels of magnesium supplementation tend to cause diarrhea, gas and bloating. Instead, supplement with chelated forms like magnesium bisglycinate, which are better absorbed by your body. Therefore, you need less than the RDA, and can avoid the unpleasant side effects.

We strongly recommend that you get more of this vital nutrient from food sources. The best food sources of magnesium are nuts, seeds, beans and brown rice.

Here are just a few of magnesium's essential functions:

- It is critical for life. One study showed that subjects who were in the highest 25% of magnesium blood levels had a 40% lower risk of dying from any cause during the study (with a 40% decrease in heart attack and stroke deaths and a 50% decrease in cancer deaths). This was compared to subjects whose magnesium levels were in the lowest 25% of the population!
- Build bones, regulate body temperature, produce proteins, and release energy stored in muscles. Because of the latter, magnesium deficiency causes muscle spasm/shortening, contributing markedly to fibromyalgia, migraines and other pain.
- Improve brain function.
- Increase heart muscle function; has been shown to improve both exercise endurance and cardiac function.
- Protect against osteoporosis.
- Lower the risk of colon cancer by 23%.
- Improve asthma.
- Decrease the frequency of migraine headaches. In fact, the quickest and most effective way to eliminate an acute migraine headache (even more effective than narcotics) is by giving 1–2 grams of magnesium sulfate intravenously over 15–20 minutes.
- Improves hyperactivity and attention deficit disorder in children.

Minerals

* Deficiency contributes to obesity by causing insulin resistance.

It is estimated that less than half of the adult US population gets even the suboptimal daily requirements.

This is a major problem. Why?

A wide range of human diseases, including cardiovascular and metabolic diseases, skeletal disorders, respiratory illness and neurologic anomalies (stress, depression and anxiety) are linked to low tissue magnesium levels.

Magnesium deficiency can induce a wide range of clinical complications, including painful muscle spasms, fibromyalgia, arrhythmia, osteoporosis and migraines.

Certain forms of magnesium are poorly absorbed, and some can have a laxative effect. A perfect multivitamin powder will contain 100 to 200 mg of bisglycinate and other chelated forms of magnesium daily.

To help boost energy and ease pain, malic acid makes magnesium even more effective. Because of labeling regulations, the malic acid will be hiding in the "other ingredients" section on a multivitamin label.

If diarrhea and cramps are not a problem, people can take up to twice this amount of magnesium. However, if you have kidney failure with a blood creatinine level over 1.6 milligrams per deciliter (mg/dL) your doctor will have properly told you to avoid potassium and magnesium.

If you get uncomfortable diarrhea from the magnesium, cut the dosage back and then slowly increase the dose as is comfortable.

BORON

Recommended daily dosage: 1-2 mg

Boron improves bone strength, especially when combined with adequate magnesium and vitamin K. It may also help mental clarity. One researcher/professor gave half his class boron and the other half placebo for the semester, and the boron group did great on the exams, while the placebo group, well, not so much.

Several studies show that low boron levels are linked to poor immune function, increased risk of mortality, osteoporosis and cognitive decline. The health benefits of boron are numerous. Boron supplements enhance the body's defense system. It improves liver metabolism to regulate blood sugar. Research also confirms that boron supplements improve bone density. Boron has also yielded positive research results in enhanced embryonic development, wound healing and cancer therapy.

Food sources of boron include fruit, avocados, legumes, coffee, tea and wine.

CHROMIUM

Recommended daily dosage: 100-200 mcg

Chromium and its natural antioxidant partner, glutathione, are critical for proper insulin function, increasing insulin sensitivity and raising healthy HDL cholesterol levels. It may also decrease many of the symptoms of low blood sugar such as getting "hangry," a form of adrenal fatigue where you get irritable when hungry and need to eat immediately.

Chromium can even be useful in depression, particularly when carbohydrate craving is a prominent symptom. A study of 113 people found that chromium supplements reduced depression-related cravings for sweets and starches and provided an overall general improvement in depressive symptoms. Some physicians think chromium also helps promote weight loss.

Chromium is one of the vital minerals involved in the prevention of cardiovascular disease (CVD) and has been shown to lower blood pressure, improve lipid metabolism, reduce inflammation and neutralize oxidative stress.

Food sources of chromium include nuts, whole grains, shellfish, broccoli, meat and wine.

COPPER

Recommended daily dosage: 500 mcg (½ mg)

Copper is a double-edged sword. Although it's critical for antioxidant production (such as SOD—superoxide dismutase—one of the body's natural free-radical scavengers that reduces pain and inflammation, as we discussed in Chapter 4), copper is also a potent free radical trigger and is quite toxic in excess.

For example, one study showed that men in the highest 25% of copper levels in their blood were 50% more likely to die during the study when compared to subjects in the lowest 25%. To strike a balance, we recommend a small dose of 500 mcg (just ½ mg) of copper each day.

Food sources of copper include shellfish, whole grains and green leafy vegetables.

IODINE

Recommended daily dosage: 100–200 mcg

Iodine is critical for both breast tissue and healthy thyroid function. Iodine deficiency (with secondary goiters) was common in the US until the food industry began to add iodine to wheat flour and salt. This eliminated much of the problem until flour makers started substituting toxic (and cheaper) bromine instead of iodine.

Iodine intake has dropped by as much as 50% in the last few decades, largely due to the change in food additives. The switch can worsen the effects of iodine deficiency, since bromine may block thyroid function.

In 2023, the Food and Drug Administration (FDA) finally officially recognized the dangers of brominated vegetable oil and has taken steps to ban the use of bromine in food.

Other minerals in the iodine family (called halides) include chloride and fluoride. Almost ubiquitous in municipal water systems, these minerals can also block iodine receptors.

Hypothyroidism (low thyroid function) is caused by iodine deficiency. It leads to a host of symptoms including not only fatigue, weight gain and pain, but also infertility and miscarriages. Low maternal iodine intake may cause hyperactivity disorder with an accompanying loss of 18 IQ score points in their children.

Research shows that women with breast cancer often have low iodine levels.

Iodine deficiency is also a common trigger for breast tenderness and fibrocystic breast disease, possible precursors to breast cancer. We suggest women who have these conditions supplement with iodine. It has even been suggested that seaweed, which is naturally high in iodine, may lower breast cancer risk.

You'll also find iodine in most types of seafood, dairy products and eggs.

MOLYBDENUM

Recommended daily dosage: 62–125 mcg

This mineral can be helpful for those with allergies, especially sulfite sensitivities (e.g. triggered by wine). It may also help detoxify acetaldehydes, which are made by yeast and may contribute to hangover.

Food sources of molybdenum include legumes, whole grains, green leafy vegetables, dairy products, beef, chicken and eggs.

SELENIUM

Recommended daily dosage: 28–55 mcg

Selenium is critical for immune function, which is important in preventing both infections and cancer.

But selenium is another "double-edged sword."

For example, three studies suggested that selenium may decrease the risk of colon cancer by about 33%. On the other hand, other research has suggested that too high selenium intake, especially in the presence of low levels of folic acid, may be associated with an increased risk of cancer.

Another concern is that increased levels of selenium were associated with increased diabetes risk (at doses over 55 mcg daily), so a great multivitamin keeps selenium levels at 55 mcg.

More is not better, but selenium is critical to health. Selenium is an important antioxidant and deficiency is associated with thyroid disease as well as other problems.

CRITICAL NUTRIENTS FOR THYROID FUNCTION

We know iodine and tyrosine are the premier nutrients for thyroid health. The key thyroid hormone, called thyroxine or T4, is simply tyrosine with four iodine atoms attached.

But we often forget that other nutrients are critical as well. These are especially important:

* Selenium. 200 mcg a day was shown to improve Hashimoto's thyroiditis. In people with this condition, selenium supplementation can be increased from 55 mcg to a total of 200 mcg daily.

* Iron. Ferritin levels under 60 ng/mL make it difficult for the body to convert T4 to its active form.

Selenium is important for antioxidant defense, formation of thyroid hormones, DNA synthesis, fertility and reproduction.

Minerals

Selenium also has a strong role in slowing the aging process, cancer prevention, improved endurance and improved muscle function.

The bottom line? During his time in medicine, Dr. Teitelbaum has spent almost 50 years weighing the research to determine how much selenium should go in a great multivitamin. His recommendation: 28–55 mcg a day.

Selenium food sources include Brazil nuts, seafood, meat and poultry.

ZINC

Recommended daily dosage: 7.5–15 mg

Zinc has been shown to be a common deficiency, and it is critical for many roles, including immune and antioxidant function.

But especially these days, a big part of the toxicity caused by chronic infections comes from zinc deficiency.

Zinc, mood and memory

Zinc may play a role in regulating the production of dopamine, the feel-good brain chemical in the brain associated with feelings of pleasure and reward. Zinc deficiency has also been linked to ADHD.

A study of seventh graders showed that adequate zinc intake improved school performance with better memory and longer attention spans. Zinc may also help people of all ages think more clearly.

ZINC DEFICIENCY AND CHRONIC INFECTIONS: A CRITICAL RELATIONSHIP

Chronic inflammation or infections can trigger massive losses of zinc in the urine, sometimes depleting zinc to the very low levels seen in a fatal zinc deficiency immune disease called *Acrodermatitis enteropathica*.

Why is this a problem?

A little-known hormone called thymulin, which is desperately dependent on zinc, is critical for the immune gland (called the thymus) to function.

Dr. Teitelbaum remembers well when the AIDS epidemic was making its debut in the late 1980s. Even early research showed that the AIDS virus caused massive zinc deficiencies along with non-detectable thymulin levels.

Interestingly, the immune deficiencies and low thymulin testing seen in early AIDS matched those seen in the severe deadly genetic zinc deficiency noted above.

It is likely that zinc deficiency caused by the AIDS virus and likely by COVID, drives long-term effects of these viral diseases and poor outcomes, a number of which could be alleviated by simply supplementing with zinc early in the infection.

Zinc is a multipurpose trace element for the human body, as it plays a crucial part in a broad range of body functions, including healthy cell growth and development, cancer prevention, metabolism, reproductive health, optimizing antioxidant function and improving cognitive and immune system function.

Zinc is found in high protein foods, especially meat, seafood and dairy products.

As with most things, we want to aim for optimal levels. Doses over 22 mg a day are okay for short-term use to boost immunity while fighting infections. But when taken daily for years, levels over this amount can lower good HDL cholesterol.

We recommend 7.5 to 15 mg of highly absorbed zinc chelate daily.

CHAPTER 8

Amino Acids and More

Amino acids are the building blocks that make up proteins. Generally speaking, Americans get enough protein in our diets. However, there are a few specific amino acids that can be very helpful when added in supplemental form.

Here are the ones we would recommend (and those we would specifically *not* recommend) in a multivitamin powder.

ARGININE

Recommended daily dosage: 0 mg

This key amino acid found in meat, beans and nuts, is another "double-edged sword."

The main concern with arginine is that it also promotes the growth of several common and often chronic viruses, so additional supplementation is not recommended.

GLYCINE

Recommended daily dosage: 195–390 mg

Glycine, found in meats, seeds, nuts and whole grains, is a key amino acid "building block" of the super important antioxidant, glutathione. It should be included in your multivitamin because generally, humans cannot make our own glycine.

Glycine generally improves health and well-being in humans and animals.

Research strongly confirms the role of supplemental glycine in the prevention of many diseases and disorders, including cardiovascular disease, several inflammatory diseases, obesity, cancer and type 2 diabetes.

Glycine can also enhance sleep quality and neurological functions.

SERINE

Recommended daily dosage: 120–240 mg

Serine, found in nuts, eggs, cheese, beans and shellfish, is also an important antioxidant, especially for its role in brain and immune function. It is also showing a lot of promise in treating and preventing type 2 diabetes by increasing insulin sensitivity. It does all this while also improving mitochondrial energy production.

TAURINE

Recommended daily dosage: 250–500 mg

Taurine, found mainly in eggs and shellfish, has been shown to increase energy and can actually be found in some energy drinks. Unfortunately, most of these "energy drinks" largely contain caffeine and sugar—which are loan sharks for energy and should be avoided. It's better to take it in your daily multivitamin powder.

But taurine's benefits are going *way* beyond getting your "Vrooom" on.

In Japan, taurine is approved for treating congestive heart failure. It works by enhancing mitochondrial energy production.

Research supports the role of taurine in protecting our mitochondrial energy furnaces and our brain cells. This is especially important given the challenges of the modern environment.

There is more. Taurine also shows benefits in optimizing blood pressure, protecting people from heart attacks and other heart damage, balancing inflammation and decreasing oxidative stress. In Japan, it has already been medically approved to treat heart failure. So, it is no surprise that it also helps stamina in general.

TYROSINE

Recommended daily dosage: 188–377 mg

Tyrosine, found in soy, nuts, avocados, dairy products and seeds, is critical for producing adrenaline and dopamine, two neurotransmitters that increase energy. That's good news for you "adrenaline junkies" out there (You know who you are!).

In simple terms, tyrosine helps your mind function better when you are under stress.

Tyrosine is also the backbone of thyroid hormone production. When you hear about the thyroid hormone thyroxine, the designation "T4" refers to tyrosine plus 4 iodine atoms. Want to give your thyroid what it needs? Iodine and tyrosine are key places to begin.

NUTRITIONAL COFACTORS

CHOLINE

Recommended daily dosage: 50–100 mg

This nutrient found in meat, eggs, poultry, fish, dairy products and cruciferous vegetables like broccoli, is critical for brain function.

Choline is required to produce acetylcholine, a neurotransmitter responsible for memory, muscle control and mood.

Decades of research have shown that choline supplements given to pregnant women produces profound benefits on their babies' brain health, cognitive function and intelligence.

Eggs are confirmed to lower the risk of dementia and Alzheimer's disease in people who eat the Standard American Diet, since egg yolks are high in choline. These benefits can also be obtained by enjoying a Mediterranean diet, especially one rich in olive oil.

MALIC ACID

Recommended daily dosage: 400-800 mg

Malic acid, found in apples, bananas, berries and a wide range of vegetables, is critical for energy production. This becomes especially important when malic acid is added to magnesium. Other side benefits? Protecting the heart muscle during heart attacks. Because of labeling regulations, its presence may be hiding in the "other ingredients" section.

BETAINE (ALSO KNOWN AS TRIMETHYLGLYCINE)

Recommended daily dosage: 175-350 mg

Betaine, found in beets, spinach and whole grains, acts as a methyl donor, meaning it helps control cell production and reproduction and even the way genes behave. This can be very helpful in energy production and for overall health. It is especially important when we think about cancer in general as the result of imperfect and/or out-of-control cell reproduction. It is an essential element in your body's ability to increase its own production of SAMe, to produce hormones in the right balance and to fight fatty liver disease, heart disease, improve body composition and help promote muscle mass and fat loss.

Betaine (although when used by itself in studies, higher doses are given) also helps lower elevated homocysteine, a compound associated with increased risk of heart attacks and stroke.

PHEW! HOW WAS THAT FOR A LOT OF INFORMATION?

But it is important to keep a sense of humor after wading through all the research... 😊

The final word on nutrition:
For those of you who watch what you eat . . . here's the final word on nutrition and health. It's a relief to know the truth after all those conflicting medical studies. They're certainly generalizations, but they are amusing:

* The Japanese eat very little fat and drink very little red wine, and they suffer fewer heart attacks than the Americans.

* The Mexicans eat a lot of fat and drink lots of Tequila and beer and they suffer fewer heart attacks than Americans.

* The French eat lots of fatty cheese and rich food and drink lots of wine, and they suffer fewer heart attacks than Americans.

* The Italians drink excessive amounts of red wine and eat lots of carbohydrate-rich pasta, and they suffer fewer heart attacks than the Americans.

* The Germans drink a lot of beers and eat lots of sausages and fats, and they suffer fewer heart attacks than the Americans.

CONCLUSION: Eat and drink what you like. Speaking English is apparently what kills you!

More helpful nutrients that we would *not* add to a multivitamin powder

This book has focused on key nutrients that *should be found in the diet but are lost in food processing,* so supplying them at the best levels in a powder as a simple and affordable daily drink is a wise choice.

There are a few other key nutrients to consider taking in addition to the vitamin powder:

Chocolate

Although supplementation with a multivitamin can be critical, there are several other wonderful ways to augment your antioxidants. This is why when Dr. Teitelbaum recommends avoiding sugar, he also adds the three magic words "except for chocolate!" Chocolate's high levels of antioxidants (especially dark chocolate) and phenolics, as well as the fact it contains a natural mood enhancer, are the reasons for this recommendation.

Chocolate has other fringe benefits. Children born to women who regularly ate chocolate during their pregnancies were more likely to be "sweet natured." Taking in high levels of antioxidants (like chocolate, but carrots and kale, too!) during pregnancy also decreases the risk of the baby having asthma. Eating chocolate is simply a sacrifice that we need to make for our children!

But chocolate does have other benefits. Eating a small square of chocolate each day was associated with a 27-45% lower risk of dying from heart attack. To put this in perspective, in people without known heart disease our interpretation of the data is that cholesterol statin medications lower heart attack deaths by only 2- 5%. And you can enjoy that time better, because eating chocolate is associated with a 70% lower risk of depression.

Red Wine

A review of 27 studies showed that drinking red wine in moderation (that means 5–12 ounces a day) can reduce the risk of heart disease and type 2 diabetes.

We don't necessarily recommend you *start* drinking for your health. But it does add more reason for those who do to enjoy it. And it goes well with chocolate!

Nutrients you shouldn't find in a vitamin powder and why

The goal of a multivitamin is to optimize the important micronutrients we should be getting from food.

While we reviewed 30 key nutrients that should be in a perfect vitamin powder, there are three important nutrients that should be left out: iron, calcium and omega fatty acids (which most people would think of as "fish oil"). Let's review these and why we feel they should not be included in multivitamins intended for everyone, and then we will discuss a few key non-dietary energy nutrients that can help fire up your body's energy furnaces.

Iron

Optimizing iron is important because an iron level that is too high or too low can cause fatigue, poor immune function, cold intolerance, decreased thyroid function, infertility and poor memory. Dr. Teitelbaum routinely recommends that people with these problems have their iron percent saturation and ferritin blood levels checked. Although the "iron level" is not useful by itself, the iron percent saturation is a useful measure and should be at least 22%. In addition, the ferritin blood level should be over 60 ng/ml.

Normal ranges of iron levels can start as low as 12 ng/ml on a ferritin blood test, a range that researchers have described as "insane." That low level will miss most people who are iron deficient and even those who have been determined to have no iron stores at all, as shown by a bone marrow biopsy.

In sick people who are anemic, some researchers even recommend keeping the ferritin above 100 ng/ml.

One study reported in the British medical journal *Lancet* showed that infertile women whose ferritin levels were between 20 and 40— remember, a ferritin level over 12 is technically normal—were often able to become pregnant only after they took supplemental iron. Other research shows that low-normal iron levels cause poor mental functioning and poor immune function. This suggests that levels considered sufficient to prevent anemia are often inadequate for other body functions.

So, the question is why not include iron in the vitamin powder?

Because "first do no harm."

One in 300 adults have a genetic iron excess called hemochromatosis. Iron supplementation can kill them. Others have a related genetic disease called thalassemia, which has similar symptoms. Most don't know that they have the disorder.

Insulin resistance, type 2 diabetes and other inflammatory conditions are often associated with excessive iron. Iron rusts, which is another way of saying that it is oxidative and can damage blood vessels and joints when levels get too high.

So, supplementing with iron is not generally recommended unless the blood test iron percent saturation is low, under 22%, or the ferritin level is under 60 ng/ml. Then supplementation using unique forms of iron that include liver fractions and ferrous bisglycinate for high absorption is suggested.

Calcium

Although companies selling calcium would have you believe that every woman should be on it, it is actually a minor player in treating osteoporosis. In fact, the countries with the highest dietary calcium intakes also have the highest levels of osteoporosis, though, to be accurate, many other factors cause bone loss, including low dietary protein and a couch potato lifestyle.

Calcium is found in abundance in dairy products and green leafy vegetables, so most of us get adequate amounts from food. Low calcium intake is not the main cause of bone density loss, and other nutrient, hormonal and lifestyle factors are much more important.

Calcium should be left out of a vitamin powder since most people do not need additional calcium, and excess calcium can block thyroid hormone absorption and may increase the risk of heart disease and other health problems if taken unnecessarily.

But the nutrients in a vitamin powder, including

vitamin D, vitamin K, magnesium, boron, and many others are far more effective at helping to build strong, healthy bones. If additional bone support is needed, add strontium 680 mg daily. Only after that should you consider adding calcium.

Omega-3 Fatty Acids

We would not add these to a multivitamin powder, because it is literally an oil from fish and oil and water don't mix.

But omega-3s are still very important for good health.

The key omega-3 essential fatty acids are eicosapentaenoic acid (EPA) and docosahexaenoic acid (DHA), the latter a major component of brain tissue. Perhaps the old wives' tales were right in calling fish "brain food!"

Even in healthy people, supplementing with omega-3s decreased anger, anxiety and depression and increased vigor. It also improves various types of attention disorders, certain cognitive and physiological functions and mood. Omega-3 fatty acids were also shown to significantly decrease stroke risk and help dry eyes.

Omega-3 fatty acids are especially important during pregnancy. Babies born to moms with high blood levels of DHA at delivery had advanced attention spans (considered an indicator of IQ in babies) well into their second year of life. Because of the mercury in fish, it is likely better to simply take mercury free omega-3 support.

High omega-3 intake during pregnancy and lactation:

* Decreases the risk of the baby being born too early or needing neonatal intensive care;

* Decreases the risk of the child getting asthma by 50%;
* Significantly decreases the risk of postpartum depression.

Nearly 60% of the brain is fat, so it is not surprising that supplemental fatty acids have been shown to be helpful in many brain processes, including depression and schizophrenia that is unresponsive to drug treatment alone. This was seen in five of six double-blind, placebo-controlled trials in schizophrenia, and four of six such trials in depression. Omega-3 EPA was also found to be beneficial in the treatment of borderline personality disorder and attention deficit hyperactivity disorder (ADHD) and is helpful in treating the depression associated with bipolar illness (manic-depressive illness).

If you have dry eyes or dry mouth, this is an indicator of omega fatty acid deficiency. If you are pregnant or nursing, have depression or have an inflammatory disease, additional omega-3 intake can be helpful. For most people, Dr. Teitelbaum recommends simply eating salmon, tuna, or sardines 3–4 times a week. However, heavy metal contamination of fatty fish like tuna is a real concern. So, if you don't eat fish, or if you are pregnant, look for omega-3s from the head of the salmon (not the oil from the body of the fish) combined with phospholipids. This form of omega-3 is very stable, with no concerns of contamination by mercury and no rancidity. So, no fish oil burps!

One More Natural Energy Maker That Is Probably Not in Your Diet

Several nutrients and herbs are especially important for making energy. We discussed B Vitamins and magnesium above, but there is one more nutrient that may not be a significant part of your diet, or that you are not getting enough of, that we need to take daily to optimize energy: coenzyme Q10.

Coenzyme Q10

Coenzyme Q10 (CoQ10) is critical for energy production.

CoQ10 is predominantly made by our bodies, with very little being present in the diet. It can become depleted during periods of excessive energy demand. Levels of CoQ10 are also significantly lower in women who use oral contraceptives or conjugated hormone replacement (Premarin and Provera are two brand names), which may in turn increase the risk of cardiovascular disease.

In addition, most cholesterol-lowering drugs deplete CoQ10. This is especially tragic because CoQ10 deficiency can cause or aggravate congestive heart failure seen in patients with heart disease-and doctors are largely unaware of this, simply blaming it on the heart disease without recognizing the underlying problem.

In addition to helping energy and heart disease, studies have demonstrated that Coenzyme Q10 can:

* Enhance immune function,

* Decrease the frequency of migraine headaches,

* Raise low sperm counts,
* Help slow Parkinson's disease,
* Improve exercise tolerance in sedentary people.

Dr. Teitelbaum takes a special form of a chewable CoQ10, 100 mg a day, that is combined with gamma cyclodextrin. This increases absorption and makes this one simple chewable equal to about 700 mg of a standard CoQ10 capsule.

PART 3

THE SOLUTION

CHAPTER 9

What Proof Do We Have?

We've heard the naysayers about the value of multivitamins. You've probably heard them too, and maybe even voiced them yourself.

What some skeptics say

We often hear arguments against multivitamins that go something like this:

1. Because many vitamins are excreted in urine, we're just making expensive urine.

2. Human beings have survived thousands of years without multivitamins.

3. Taking supplements is unscientific, as *they* have seen no research showing that they help.

Let's start by addressing these points. Then we can move forward with what the science actually shows.

Expensive urine

We think the skeptics are making an excellent case, and

they should demonstrate how strong their belief is by following their own advice.

Water simply goes out in their urine, so we propose the skeptics stop drinking. Then they can stop annoying people who are endeavoring to improve their health. We're a little tongue in cheek here, but you get the point and the ridiculousness of this viewpoint.

Human beings have survived thousands of years without multivitamins

That's true! Human beings have also survived thousands of years without the extensive food processing that has infiltrated almost all our food supply. Add in the depleted soil nutrients due to factory farming, plus the insecticides and pesticides added to crops, and we have the makings for an epidemic of vitamin and mineral deficiencies.

But it gets worse.

Today, the average American gets more than one-third of their daily calories from sugar and white flour, which have almost no nutritional value, are chock full of empty calories and have most of the vitamins and minerals removed.

Today, much of our food is trucked hundreds, even thousands of miles, sometimes losing its nutritional value with every mile.

Our ancestors grew or foraged or hunted what they ate. Their diet was natural and fresh and consumed almost immediately.

By contrast, today's humans live in a nutritional desert.

A study in the *American Journal of Clinical Nutrition* showed that fewer than 5% of the study participants consumed even the government's woefully low recommended daily amounts (RDAs) of all their needed vitamins and minerals. What is frightening is that this study was conducted in Beltsville, Maryland, on U.S. Department of Agriculture (USDA) research center employees!

We went into this in detail in Chapter 2, so we won't re-hash it, but we'll just leave you with the idea that some people think, without evidence, that we don't need multivitamins because our food should be enough. It's not enough. Not anymore. Period.

Taking supplements is unscientific, as they have seen no research showing that supplements improve health.

That's just not true. There are thousands of studies on the value of multivitamins and on vitamin, mineral and amino acid supplements. Yes, we'll admit, the evidence is mixed, but we can say, unequivocally that our combined decades of experience in this field holds true:

Multivitamins make a big difference.

No, multivitamins cannot and should not substitute for a healthy diet rich in whole grains, fresh vegetables and fruits, lean proteins and healthy fats. But the evidence is there, if you choose to read just 4,675 studies posted on the National Library of Medicine's PubMed research database under the search term "multivitamins." Add in another 461 on the "benefits of multivitamins" and 24,463 results for "benefits of supplements." That doesn't even include the research into individual vitamins, minerals and other nutrients discussed in this book. Just for the sake of argument, searching PubMed for "benefits of vitamin C" gives you 2,308 published studies as of this writing.

We're guessing you probably don't want to read 30,000 or more journal articles. We surely don't blame you! That's why we've extracted a sampling of the most important ones in our reference section at the end of this book.

We've mentioned some of the research on the value of multivitamins in the preceding three chapters. We've also included warnings about what not to take, as well as warnings about maximum dosages and potential for harm from incorrect dosages of certain nutrients. In a high-quality multivitamin, these are all taken into account. The two of us have spent many decades investigating the vitamins, minerals, aminos and other nutrients we've discussed here.

Yes, there are some bad actors out there. There are unscrupulous companies that market fakes or even add ingredients, including pharmaceuticals, that can be harmful. In the next chapter, we hope to give you the tools to determine what's essential, what's good and what's bad.

Read on . . .

CHAPTER 10

The Right Stuff

We'll be the first to admit that this part is a bit of a slog. That's because the government prohibits us from recommending a specific product. That puts the burden on you to find The Right Stuff in your multivitamin. We're here to make it as simple as possible. We regret that you'll have to do some of the work yourself.

Being science geeks, we have carefully evaluated thousands of studies showing the benefits of natural therapies, especially the value of nutrients. We are both saddened by how depleted the American diet is and how great is the need for supplementation just to prevent serious disease, loss of vitality and premature aging caused by nutritional deficiencies.

There are countless other herbal and nutritional treatments that are enormously helpful. Even the best multivitamin is not meant to replace all of these. But rather it is meant to be the foundation and starting point for vibrant health and vitality.

Our goal? Supply *optimal* levels of the key nutrients that should be found in the diet, which are nowadays horribly deficient.

So that's what we did.

We sat down and determined what humans need, the most effective levels of each of the dietary micronutrients, including vitamins, minerals, key amino acids and key energy cofactors.

This ideal micronutrient list totals about 7,000 mg of nutrients daily.

Even if you could squeeze those nutrients into 500 mg capsules, excuse us, horse pills, presuming no binders or fillers, that would take 14 capsules a day! In real life, the total turns out to be closer to 30-50 capsules a day.

That's simply not something most people will or should do.

Then came an "aha—Eureka!" moment. What if these were all put together in a good tasting powder? Then people could just add it to water, juice or a smoothie and optimize their nutrition with one easy, tasty and affordable drink each day.

Other Benefits

Looking at the powder further, it became more and more clear that this is a wonderful way to help people thrive in a modern environment.

Such a great multivitamin:

* Improves compliance, because it's easy to take each morning;

* Is much more cost effective to make and considerably less expensive for you to buy. You'd be surprised at how much it costs to make pills, containers and all the different things that go along with packaging and

marketing 30 separate supplements. Making it with a powder not only makes it easier to take, but dramatically lowers cost;

* Can be adjusted easily for sensitive stomachs and systems.

Sometimes starting with a full dose is too powerful and can overstimulate the gut. If this is a problem, powders can be easily adjusted. Start with a quarter scoop daily and work up over time to what feels best. One-half to one scoop a day of the best multivitamin powder would each give powerful nutritional support.

The Right Stuff

Next comes the choice of the best forms of different nutrients. Splurge when it is helpful and worth *your* while, instead of wasting your money on what is simply trendy and expensive, but not especially beneficial. Nix on those endless TV commercials touting various magical vitamin combos!

Creating a great multivitamin means being picky about the forms of the nutrients used. For example, the perfect multi should include a range of vitamin E tocopherols, the 5 MTHF form of folate and the retinol form of vitamin A. The list goes on.

So much of marketing gears to what is trendy instead of truly beneficial. So, part of our role as experts is to help pick what gives *you* the most bang for the buck.

Basically, the best multivitamin powder will have *The Right Stuff!*

The Importance of Being Methylation Friendly

Have you been exhausted for years? Brain fog? Generalized pain? Can't sleep? Have you had COVID or been diagnosed with chronic fatigue or fibromyalgia? Maybe you think it's just a sign of aging.

It could be many things, but it's worth considering that you may have a methylation problem. This complex chemical process, which often follows a serious infection, is critical for hundreds of important biochemical reactions in the body, especially in the making of energy and the antioxidant glutathione.

It becomes a problem when your body attempts to shut down energy production to conserve energy or to starve infections.

Sometimes this methylation process gets stuck and can't turn back on when the infection passes. This can leave you stranded in a cycle of exhaustion and unable to use nutrients to make energy efficiently.

But there is a trick. Several vitamins and nutrients help bypass this methylation blockade, making them "methylation friendly." Again, this includes picking *the right stuff.*

A great vitamin powder would take methylation needs and all the above into account, adding nutrients such as 5-MTHF, betaine (trimethylglycine), and methylcobalamin. These are a bit pricier to use than the standard forms of nutrients, but well worth it!

DOES DR. TEITELBAUM RECOMMEND GENETIC METHYLATION TESTING? NOPE!

Genetic testing for methylation deficiencies is not helpful, so don't bother with it.

Since most of the population has at least some deviation from "standard," it's not going to add any helpful information in terms of treatment. Normal differences are being called genetic "defects" when they are often simply meaningless variations.

So yes, as nice as it is to have a positive test to explain your CFS/fibromyalgia or long COVID, methylation testing (called MTHFR or other tests that are positive in virtually everybody— healthy or not), may not be the best way to go.

Instead of testing, I find it best to simply have your multivitamin be methylation friendly, i.e. the multivitamin that turns back on the body functions impaired by an infection. That automatically takes care of the problem and you don't have to worry about the details.

PS: For more on methylation and how to recover from CFS and fibromyalgia, I invite you to read my book *From Fatigued to Fantastic*. For long COVID, I recommend my book *You Can Heal from Long Covid*.

I have been the principal investigator on eight studies showing effective treatments for these conditions, and these books summarize what I have learned about effective treatment for chronic fatigue, CFS, fibromyalgia and long Covid.

Here's the formula we suggest:

Vitamin / Mineral / Amino Acid	Amt/serving
Vitamin A (as retinyl palmitate)	1,500 mcg (5,000 IU)
Vitamin C (from calcium ascorbate)	250 mg
Vitamin D3 (as cholecalciferol)	25 mcg (1,000 IU)
Vitamin E (as d-alpha and mixed tocopherols)	50 mg (75 IU)
Thiamin (Vitamin B1) (from thiamin HCl)	50 mg
Riboflavin (Vitamin B2)	75 mg
Niacin (Vitamin B3) (as niacin and from niacinamide)	50 mg
Vitamin B6 (from pyridoxal-5-phosphate)	25 mg
Folate (from calcium-l-5-methyltetrahydrofolate)	340 mcg DFE
Vitamin B12 (as methylcobalamin)	500 mcg
Biotin (as d-biotin)	200 mcg
Pantothenic acid (from d-calcium pantothenate)	100 mg
Choline (from choline bitartrate)	100 mg
Calcium (from dicalcium phosphate calcium fructoborate, d-calcium pantothenate, and calcium ascorbate)	75 mg
Iodine (from potassium iodide)	200 mcg
Magnesium (magnesium bisglycinate chelate)	200 mg
Zinc (from zinc bisglycinate chelate)	15 mg

The Right Stuff

Vitamin / Mineral / Amino Acid	Amt/serving
Selenium (from selenium yeast) (Saccharomyces cerevisiae)	55 mcg
Copper (from copper glycinate chelate)	0.5 mg
Manganese (from manganese bisglycinate chelate)	2 mg
Chromium (from chromium nicotinate glycinate chelate)	200 mcg
Molybdenum (from molybdenum glycinate chelate)	125 mcg
L-Taurine	500 mg
L-Glycine	390 mg
L-Tyrosine	377 mg
Betaine Anhydrous	350 mg
N-Acetyl-L-Cysteine	250 mg
L-Serine	240 mg
Boron (from calcium fructoborate)	2 mg
Vitamin K2 (as menaquinone-7)	100 mcg

> **WHAT DR. TEITELBAUM TAKES EACH DAY**
>
> * The perfect vitamin powder;
> * One vectorized omega-3 with phospholipids;
> * CoQ10 100 mg (a chewable with gamma cyclodextrin);
> * A unique, highly absorbed curcumin with turmeric essential oils, 750 mg daily.
>
> This vitamin powder and 3 tablets or capsules replaces over 60 pills each day. And I feel fantastic!

In conclusion . . .

As we mentioned in earlier chapters, a high-quality multivitamin gives you the most effective dosage of vitamins, minerals and amino acids for good health. But, as we're sure you are aware, many of us have a host of other health challenges that will benefit from a wide variety of other nutrients and botanicals.

You've noticed that Dr. Teitelbaum takes curcumin and Terry takes a fairly broad variety of botanicals each day in addition to the perfect multivitamin powder to address specific health conditions as well as general well-being.

The perfect multivitamin lays a powerful and easy foundation for overall health and vitality. It's an excellent "Step 1" for your nutritional support program!

References

NOTE: This is a very tiny sampling of study references. There are many hundreds.

Chapter 1: Why Do You Need a Multivitamin?

R.M. Marston and B.B. Peterkin. Nutrient Content of the National Food Supply, *National Food Review*, 1980 Winter, 21–25.

H.A. Schroeder. Losses of Vitamins and Trace Minerals Resulting from Processing and Preservation of Foods. *Am J Clin Nutr.* 1971 May;24(5): 562–573.

H.C. Trowell, ed.. Western Diseases: Their Emergence and Prevention. Cambridge, MA, Harvard University Press, 1981.

Mertz W, ed.. Beltsville 1 Year Dietary Intake Survey. *Am J Clin Nutr.* 1984 Dec.;40, supplement:1323–1403.

Bartali B et al. Low Micronutrient Levels as a Predictor of Incident Disability in Older Women. *Arch Intern Med.* 006;166:2335–2340.

Marniemi J. Dietary and Serum Vitamins and Minerals as Predictors of Myocardial Infarction and Stroke in Elderly Subjects. *Nutr Metab Cardiovasc Dis.* 2005 Jun;15(3):188–97. 43761 (10/2005).

COSMOS Studies: Multivitamin Associated with 2–3 Year Lower Brain Age. https://ajcn.nutrition.org/article/S0002-9165(23)48904-6/fulltext

Vyas CN, Manson JE et al. Effect of Multivitamin-Mineral Supplementation Versus Placebo on Cognitive Function: Results from the Clinic Subcohort of the COcoa Supplement and Multivitamin Outcomes Study (COSMOS) randomized clinical trial and meta-analysis of 3 cognitive studies within COSMOS. *Am. J Clin. Nutr.* 2024 Mar.; 119;692–701.

WHAT PROOF DO WE HAVE? SPECIFIC NUTRIENTS

Antioxidants

Kennes B, Dumont et al. Effect of Vitamin C Supplements on Cell-Mediated Immunity in Old People. *Gerontology* 1983;29:305–310.

Chandra RK. Effect of Macro and Micronutrient Deficiencies and Excess on Immune Response, *Food Technology*, February 1985, pp. 91–93.

Chandra S, et al.. Undernutrition Impairs Immunity. *Internal Medicine.* 1985 Dec;5: 85–99.

Litonjua AA, Rifas-Shiman SL, et al. Maternal Antioxidant Intake in Pregnancy and Wheezing Illnesses in Children at 2 Y of Age. *Am J Clin Nutr.* 2006;84(4):903–11.

van Leeuwen R, Boekhoorn S, et al. Dietary Intake of Antioxidants and Risk of Age-related Macular Degeneration. *JAMA.* 2005; 294(24): 3101–7.

Kwun IS, Park KH, et al. Lower Antioxidant Vitamins (A, C and E) and Trace Minerals (Zn, Cu, Mn, Fe and Se) Status with Cerebrovascular Disease. *Nutr Neurosci.* 2005;8(4):251–7.)

Yesilbursa D, Serdar A, et al. Effect of N-acetylcysteine on Oxidative Stress and Ventricular Function in Myocardial Infarction, *Heart Vessels*, 2006;21(1):33–7.

Lafleur DL, Pittenger C, et al.. N-acetylcysteine augmentation in Serotonin Reuptake Inhibitor Refractory Obsessive-Compulsive Disorder. *Psychopharmacology.* 2006 Jan.;184(2):254–6.)

Vitamins

Vitamin C

Das S, Ray R, et al. Effect of Ascorbic Acid on Prevention of Hypercholesterolemia Induced Atherosclerosis. *Mol Cell Biochem.* 2006 Feb 14.

Sasazuki S, Sasaki S, et al. Effects of Vitamin C on Common Cold: Randomized Controlled Trial. *Eur J Clin Nutr.* 2005 Aug. 24.

Sylvester PW, Shah SJ. Mechanisms Mediating the Antiproliferative and Apoptotic Effects of Vitamin E in Mammary Cancer Cells. *Front Biosci.* 2005 Jan 1;10:699–709.

References

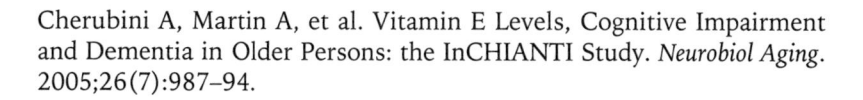

Cherubini A, Martin A, et al. Vitamin E Levels, Cognitive Impairment and Dementia in Older Persons: the InCHIANTI Study. *Neurobiol Aging.* 2005;26(7):987–94.

Vitamin A

Ray AL, Semba RD, et al. Low Serum Selenium and Total Carotenoids Predict Mortality among Older Women: The Women's Health and Aging Studies. *J Nutr.* 2006;136(1):172–6.

Huang, J., et al. Association Between Serum Retinol and Overall and Cause-specific Mortality in a 30-year Prospective Cohort Study. *Nat Commun.* 2021;12:6418.

Vitamin B1 (Thiamine)

Hanninen SA, Darling PB, et al. The Prevalence of Thiamin Deficiency in Hospitalized with CHF. *J Am Coll Cardiol.* 2006;47(2):354–61.

Gold M. Plasma and Red Blood Cell Thiamin Deficiency in Patients with Dementia of the Alzheimer's Type. *Arch Neurol.* 1995 Nov.;52(11):1081–1086. #23739.

Vitamin B6 (pyridoxine)

Lin PT, Cheng CH, et al. Low Pyridoxal 5' Phosphate is Associated with Increased Risk of Coronary Artery Disease. *Nutrition.* 2006 Oct 9. [Epub ahead of print].

Vitamin B12 (Methylcobalamin)

J. Lindenbaum, et al. Neuropsychiatric Disorders by Cobalamin Deficiency in the Absence of Anemia. *N Engl J Med.* 1988 June 30;318(26):1720–1728.

W.S. Beck, Cobalamin and the Nervous System, editorial. *N Engl J Med.* 1988 June 30;318(26): 1752–1754.

Lindenbaum J, Rosenberg IH et al. Prevalence of Cobalamin Deficiency in the Framingham Elderly Population. *Am J Clin Nutr.* 1994 July;60(1): 2–11.

Folate

Ravaglia G, Forti P, et al. Homocysteine and Folate as Risk Factors for Dementia and Alzheimer's Disease, *Am J Clin Nutr.* 2005;82(3);636–43.

Wang Y, et al. Folic Acid in Patients with Cardiovascular Disease: A Meta-analysis. *Medicine.* 2019 Sep;98(37):e17095.

Vitamin D

Holick MF. High Prevalence of Vitamin D Inadequacy and Implications for Health. *Mayo Clin Proc.* 2006;81(3):353–73.

Vitamin K

DiNicolantonio JJ, et al. The Health Benefits of Vitamin K. *Open Heart.* 2015 Oct 6;2(1):e000300.

Amiri SV, et al. Does Vitamin K Improve Vitamin K Antagonist Therapy? *J Cardiol Cases.* 2022 Jan13;25(6):359–362.

Minerals

Magnesium

Seelig, MS. The Requirement of Magnesium by the Normal Adult. *Am J Clin Nutr.* 1964 June; 14:342–390.

Leone N and, D Courbon. Zinc, Copper, and Magnesium and Risks for Allcause, Cancer, and Cardiovascular mortality. *Epidemiology.* 2006;17(3):308–14.

Vinceti M, et al. Selenium Exposure and the Risk of Type 2 Diabetes: A Meta-analysis. *Eur J Epidemiol.* 2018 Sep;33(9):789–810. Epub 2018 Jul 5. PMID: 29974401.

Ray AL, et al. Low Serum Selenium and Total Carotenoids Predict Mortality among Older Women: The Women's Health and Aging Studies, *J Nutr.* 2006;136(1):172–6.

Zinc

Kiouri DP, et al. Multifunctional Role of Zinc in Human Health: An Update. *EXCLI J.* 2023 Aug 4;22:809–827.

Amino Acids

Serine

Holm LJ and KL Buschard. A Neglected Amino aAcid with a Potential Therapeutic Role in Diabetes. *APMIS.* 2019 Oct;127(10):655–659.

Index

A

acetaldehydes, 52
acetaminophen, 27
acetylcholine, 34, 36, 62
acid blockers, 38–39
acne, 32
Acrodermatitis enteropathica, 56
adrenal glands, 35, 36, 50
adrenaline, 61
aging, 25, 26, 27, 55
AIDS, 56
allergies, 53
Alzheimer's disease, 34–35, 38, 62
amino acids, 20, 21, 28, 59–62
anemia, 67
anger, 69
angina, 30
antioxidants, 25–32, 51, 54, 56, 60, 65
anxiety, 69
arginine, 59
asthma, 43, 48, 65, 70
attention deficit-hyperactivity disorder (ADHD), 48, 52, 54, 69, 70
attention spans, 55, 69

B

behavior, 34
Benton, David, 34
beta carotene, 32
betaine, 63, 82
bioindividuality, 19
biotin. *See* vitamin B7
bipolar illness, 70
birth defects, 32, 37
blood pressure, 38, 43, 46, 50, 61
blood sugar, 50
blood vessels, 27, 35, 44, 68
body fat, 30
body temperature, 48
bones, 29, 38, 43, 44, 46, 48, 50, 68–69
borderline personality disorder, 70
boron, 46, 50, 69
brain, 27, 33, 37, 48, 60, 61, 62, 69, 70
breasts, 52, 53
bromine, 52

C

calcium, 6, 22, 46, 68–69

calories, 7
cancer, 27, 32, 41, 44, 48, 54, 55, 56, 60
   breast, 31, 38, 42, 52, 53
   colon, 36, 42, 48, 53
   ovarian, 38
   prostate, 31
   skin, 42
   stomach, 29
cancer therapy, 50
carbohydrates, 51
cardiovascular disease (CVD). *See* heart disease
cells, 56, 63
   blood, 35, 37
   brain, 61
   division, 27, 63
   reproduction, 63
cheese, 46
chloride, 52
chocolate, 65–66
cholecalciferol. *See* vitamin D
cholesterol, 71
   HDL, 50, 57
choline, 62
chromium, 50–51
chronic fatigue syndrome (CFS), 82
cobalamin. *See* vitamin B12
coenzyme Q10 (CoQ10), 71–72, 86
cognition, 31, 35, 50, 55, 56, 62, 69
cold intolerance, 66
colds, 30
congestive heart failure (CHF). *See* heart disease
copper, 27, 51
CoQ10. *See* coenzyme Q10 (CoQ10)
Coumadin, 44
COVID, 56, 83
creatinine, 49
crops, 5–6, 17
curcumin, 86
cystic fibrosis, 27

D

dairy products, 46
deaths, 29, 32, 48, 50, 51
dementia, 31, 39, 44, 62
depression, 38, 51, 66, 69, 70
   postpartum, 34, 70
detoxification, 27, 36, 37
diabetes, 27, 35, 43, 54
   Type 2, 60, 66, 68
diets, 3–4, 46, 64, 76, 77
   Mediterranean, 62
   Standard American (SAD), 7, 11, 13, 45–46, 62
   vegan, 38
digestive enzymes, 22
DNA, 54
docosahexaenoic acid (DHA), 69
dopamine, 55, 61
dry mouth, 70

E

eggs, 62
eicosapentaenoic acid (EPA), 69, 70
embryos, 50

Index

endurance, 48, 55, 61
energy, 34, 37, 38, 39, 48, 61, 62, 63, 69, 71, 82
energy drinks, 61
environmental toxins, 25
EuroPharma, 11
exercise, 72
eyes, 27, 29
   dry, 69, 70

F
farming, 5
fatigue, 39, 66, 82
fatty liver disease, 27, 63
ferritin, 54, 67, 68
ferrous bisglycinate, 68
fertility, 54, 66, 67
fibromyalgia, 48, 83
fish, 69, 70
fish oil. *See* Omega-3 fatty acids
5-methyltetrahydrofolate (5-MTHF), 37, 82
flour, 37, 52, 76
fluoride, 52
flushing, 35
folate. *See* vitamin B9
folic acid. *See* vitamin B9
foods, 3–4, 13–16, 76–77
   fast, 13–14, 16
food processing, 5, 6–7, 39, 45, 46, 47, 76
free radical oxygen species (ROS). *See* free radicals
free radicals, 25, 51
fruits, 17

G
gamma cyclodextrin, 72, 86
Giovannucci, Edward, 42
glutathione, 26–27, 28, 50, 60, 82
glycine, 28, 60
goiters, 52
Gold, Michael, 34

H
hair, 36
halides, 52
hangovers, 53
Hashimoto's thyroiditis, 54
hearing, 29
heart, 33, 46, 48, 63
heart attacks, 44, 48, 61, 63, 64, 65
heart disease, 33, 36, 43, 51, 60, 61, 63, 66, 68, 71
hemochromatosis, 67
herbicides, 6
hips, 29, 43
holistic medicine, 9–10
homocysteine, 63
hormone replacement, 71
hormones, 63
   See also thyroxine (T4)
hypothyroidism, 52

I
immune system, 7, 25–26, 32, 36, 37, 43, 50, 53, 56, 57, 60, 66, 71
indigestion, 39
infections, 55, 56

inflammation, 27, 51, 56, 60, 61, 68
inflammatory bowel disease, 43
insecticides, 76
insulin, 16, 27, 44, 50, 60
insulin resistance, 49, 68
iodine, 46, 52–53, 54, 62
iron, 6, 22, 54, 66–68

J
joints, 68

K
kidneys, 49

L
learning disorders, 34
leptin, 15
liver, 27, 35, 29, 50
liver fractions, 68
longevity, 4–5

M
magnesium, 23, 46, 47–49, 50, 63, 69
magnesium bisglycinate, 47, 49
malic acid, 49, 63
melanomas, 42
memory, 34, 36, 38, 55, 62, 66
menaquinone. *See* vitamin K
menstruation, 31
mercury, 69, 70
metabolism, 35, 51, 56
metformin, 39

methylation, 82, 83
methylation testing (MTHF), 83
methylcobalamin. *See* vitamin B12
migraines, 32, 44, 48, 71
minerals, 20, 21, 45–57
mitochondria, 60, 61
molybdenum, 53
moods, 34, 62, 65, 69
multiple sclerosis, 43
multivitamin powder, 22, 28, 49, 66, 69, 80–82, 84–86
   contents and dosages chart, 84–85
   not to be included, 22, 45–46, 59, 66–70
multivitamins, 3, 13, 17, 20, 22, 75–78, 86
muscles, 28, 48, 55, 62, 63

N
n-acetyl cysteine (NAC), 28
nails, 36
neurology, 44, 60
neuropathy, 36, 44
neurotransmitters, 61, 62
niacin. *See* vitamin B3
niacinamide, 35
nutrients, 5–7, 15, 17, 18, 19–22, 23

O
obesity, 7, 14–15, 49, 60
obsessive compulsive disorder (OCD), 28
olive oil, 62

Index

Omega fatty acids, 22
Omega-3 fatty acids, 69–70, 86
oral contraceptives, 71
osteoporosis, 30, 32, 39, 43, 46, 48, 50, 68
oxidation, 26, 68
　fat, 30
oxidative stress, 51, 61
oxygen, 25

P
pancreas, 16
pantothenic acid. *See* vitamin B5
Parkinson's disease, 27, 44, 72
pesticides, 6, 76
phenolics, 65
phospholipids, 70, 86
phosphorus, 5, 6
potassium, 46, 49
pregnancies, 37, 62, 65, 67, 69
protein pump inhibitors (PPIs), 38–39
proteins, 48
pyridoxal-5-phosphate (P-5-P), 36
pyridoxine. *See* vitamin B6

R
Recommended Dietary Allowances (RDAs), 19–20, 22, 33, 47, 77
reproduction, 54, 56
retinol, 32
rheumatoid arthritis, 27, 43

riboflavin. *See* vitamin B2

S
salt. *See* sodium
SAMe, 63
schizophrenia, 70
scurvy, 20, 29
sea salt, 46
seaweed, 53
selenium, 53–55
serine, 60
skin, 32, 35, 36
sleep, 39, 50
smoothies, 18
SOD. *See* super oxide dismutase (SOD)
sodium, 46, 52
soil depletion, 5–6, 17, 76
sperm, 30, 72
statins, 65–66
stomach acid, 39
stress, 8–9, 39, 62
strokes, 29, 30, 38, 48, 63, 69
strontium 680, 69
sudden infant death syndrome (SIDS), 34
sugar, 7, 76
sulfites, 53
sulfur, 5
sun exposure, 41–42
super oxide dismutase (SOD), 27–28, 51

T
taurine, 61
Terry Naturally, 11
T4. *See* thyroxine (T4)

thalassemia, 67
thiamine. *See* vitamin B1
thymulin, 56
thymus, 56
thyroid, 46, 52, 54, 62, 66, 68
thyroxine (T4), 46, 54, 62
tocopherols, 30–31
trimethylglycine. *See* betaine
turmeric essential oils, 86
Tylenol. *See* acetaminophen
tyrosine, 54, 61–62

U
ulcerative colitis, 27

V
vascular disease, 36
vegetable oil, 52
vegetables, 17
viruses, 59
vitamin A, 32
vitamin B1, 33–34
vitamin B2, 6, 34
vitamin B3, 34–35
vitamin B5, 35–36
vitamin B6, 36
vitamin B7, 36
vitamin B9, 37, 54
vitamin B12, 38–39, 38, 82
vitamin C, 6, 20, 21, 29–30
vitamin D, 41–43, 46, 69
vitamin E, 28, 30–31
vitamin K, 43–44, 50, 69
vitamins, 20, 21, 29–39, 41–44, 75
   See also multivitamin powder; multivitamins
Vito, Ed, 10–11

W
water systems, 52
weight loss, 51, 63
wine
   red, 66
wound healing, 50

Y
yeast, 7, 53

Z
zinc, 27, 32, 55–57

About the Authors

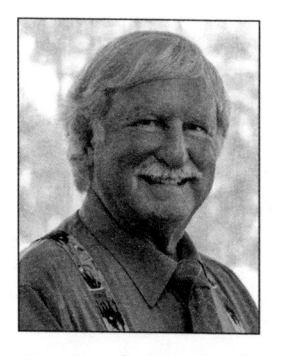

Jacob Teitelbaum, M.D., is one of the most frequently quoted integrative medical authorities in the world. He is the author of 12 books, including the best-selling *You Can Heal From Long COVID, From Fatigued to Fantastic!, Pain Free, 1,2,3!, The Fatigue and Fibromyalgia Solution* and *Diabetes Is Optional.* He is the lead author of eight studies on effective treatment for fibromyalgia and chronic fatigue syndrome, and the popular Cures A-Z phone app. Learn more at www.Vitality101.com. Questions? Contact him at FatigueDoc@gmail.com.

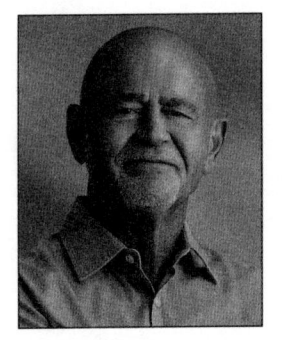

Terry Lemerond is a natural health expert with over 55 years of experience. He has owned health food stores, founded dietary supplement companies, and formulated over 500 products.

A much sought-after speaker and accomplished author, Terry shares his wealth of experience and knowledge in health and nutrition through social media, newsletters, podcasts, webinars, and personal speaking engagements. His books include *Seven Keys to Vibrant Health* and the sequel, *Seven Keys to Unlimited Personal Achievement,* and his newest publication, *50+ Natural Health Secrets Proven to Change Your Life.* His continual dedication, energy and zeal are part of his ongoing mission to improve the health of America.

KNOWLEDGE IS POWER,
ESPECIALLY FOR YOUR HEALTH!

Are you in search of a reliable, science-based resource for all your health and nutrition questions? Terry Talks Nutrition has you covered.

Connect with Terry to increase your knowledge on a wide variety of topics, including immunity, pain, curcumin and cancer, diabetes, and so much more!

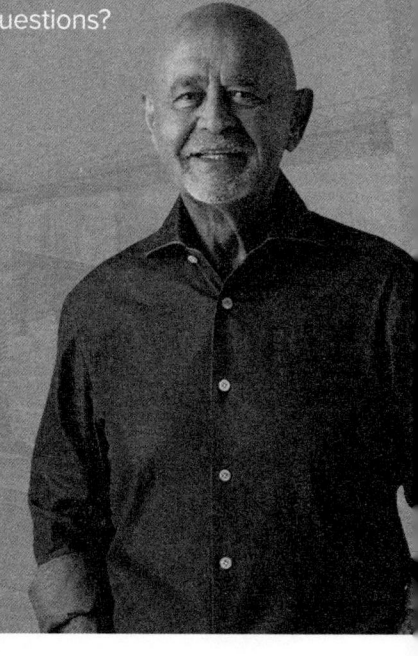

READ
Visit TerryTalksNutrition.com for today's latest and greatest health and nutrition information.

LISTEN
Tune in on Sat. and Sun. 8-9 am (CST) at TerryTalksNutrition.com for a live internet radio show hosted by Terry! You can listen to past shows on the website or on your favorite podcast app.

ENGAGE
Connect with us on Facebook, where you can engage with other individuals seeking safe and effective ways to improve overall wellness.

WATCH
Check out our educational YouTube Channel to learn from the world's leading doctors and health experts.

Simply open your smartphone camera. Hold over desired code above for more information.

Get answers to all of your health questions at **TERRYTALKSNUTRITION.COM**

WELCOME TO
ttn publishing

Are you ready to learn how anyone can use natural medicines, safely and effectively, to improve their health? You'll love TTN Publishing, my newest endeavor to bring you cutting edge research on powerful, health-supporting botanicals. I've coauthored numerous books with top alternative doctors from around the world to help you learn all you can about taking your health into your own hands. These educational books, supported by powerful scientific research, contain all the information you need to live a life of vibrant health.

In Good Health,
Terry Lemerond

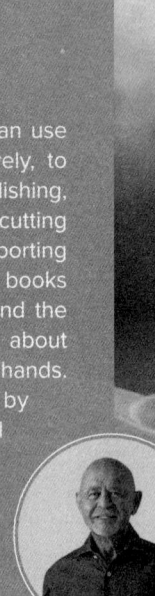

ADDITIONAL BOOKS BY TTN PUBLISHING:

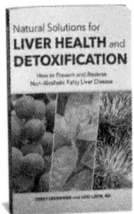

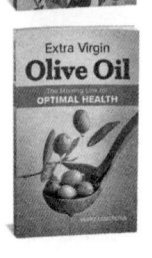

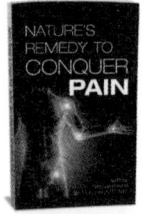

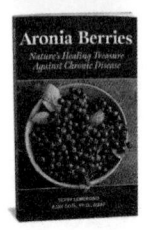

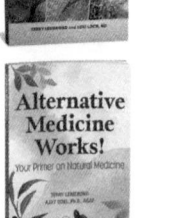

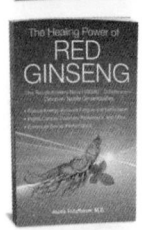

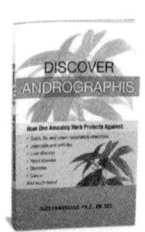

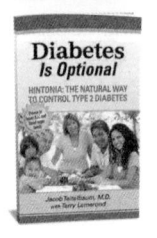

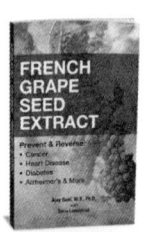

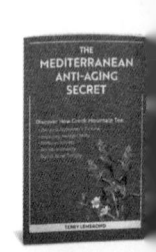

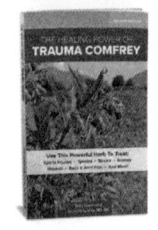

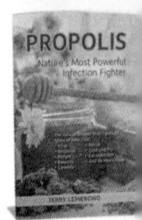

- Natural Solutions for LIVER HEALTH and DETOXIFICATION
- NATURE'S REMEDY TO CONQUER PAIN
- DISCOVER ANDROGRAPHIS
- FRENCH GRAPE SEED EXTRACT
- THE MEDITERRANEAN ANTI-AGING SECRET
- Alternative Medicine Works!
- The Healing Power of RED GINSENG
- Diabetes Is Optional
- THE HEALING POWER OF TRAUMA COMFREY
- PROPOLIS
- Extra Virgin Olive Oil
- Aronia Berries

Get a copy for yourself and gift them to the people you care about!

©2024_09_EP